Advance Praise

"*Brilliant Burnout* is an innovative and extremely captivating guide for women wanting to reclaim their power and take control of their burnout. Through her remarkable multifaceted approach to balancing women's hormones and health, Nisha Jackson is successful in helping women break through and reinvent their physical, emotional, and mental health, just when they might have thought they couldn't feel great again! Rare, indeed, is the medical practitioner today that can combine a deep understanding of women's health, years of clinical expertise, and real patient insights from over 25 years in the field all in one book.

I have seen firsthand the epidemic of modern-day women who are burning out and wondering why. Is this how life is going to be from here on out? *Brilliant Burnout* is the ultimate wake-up call for women who no longer choose to tolerate feeling terrible. In it, Nisha shares insight for those dying to know the secrets behind how the most successful and brilliant women are using their hormonal systems to harness their health. Nisha is a groundbreaking author in the field of medicine, and she finally created a book that shows how hormones are essential for balance but are only part of the entire equation for the modern-day brilliant woman looking to achieve ultimate and lasting energy and longevity. This book showcases and solidifies Nisha Jackson as a true expert in her field and offers women accurate and invaluable advice with real solutions so that they can finally get back to how they used to feel, with beauty, grace, and power.

This book includes real-life examples of how devastating hormone imbalance can be for women, which I have spent my entire life researching, training, and sharing with other practitioners and physicians. Nisha Jackson is a progressive hormone expert and a huge advocate for strong women today who believes in helping all women achieve more while staying balanced, happy, and healthy. All of this is possible with the right steps and recalibration of the brain, body, and hormones. It is the only way to regain health and wellness. *Brilliant Burnout* has paved the way for women all over the world to finally get back to their brilliance!"

—Neal Rouzier, MD, director of The Preventative Medicine Clinic, worldwide recognized speaker and expert on h̶ renown

D1221992

"Once again, Dr. Jackson has hit it out of the ballpark with her latest book, *Brilliant Burnout*. In it, she describes very accurately all the stages of adrenal stress, exhaustion, and burnout, as well as the interactions involved in the stress response between the adrenals, ovaries, and other endocrine organs such as the thyroid, pituitary, hypothalamus, and the brain. This is a handbook for any woman who isn't feeling her best but doesn't know how to pinpoint the problem. It is also an excellent resource for any healthcare practitioner who needs a well-organized, in-depth resource on tips to diagnose and treat health challenges that have chronically high levels of stress as the basis for development. Readers can quickly determine which chapter (or chapters) are pertinent to their current situation by scanning questions at the beginning of each chapter and, if need be, reviewing the lists ending each chapter, which detail action steps that should be taken to enable the body to heal, repair, and recover from the 12 stages of burnout. I only wish this book had been available 20 years ago!"

—**E. Stroud,** RN, BSN Talent, Oregon

"Nisha Jackson has mastered her practice as a medical and hormone expert, and her book, *Brilliant Burnout*, is the ultimate guide for women to not only stay hormonally balanced and energized but also live a happy and successful life!"

—**Jennifer Sullivan,** CEO, owner, and inventor of the female-owned business Guzzle Buddy

"I have been privileged to work with Nisha for over a decade. Never one to accept the status quo, she is a tireless advocate for her patients. She has a passion for life and learning that is contagious, and she has inspired countless women to challenge themselves to become better people, myself included. Her new book is yet another testament to her continued devotion to finding the best treatments to promote health and wellness."

—**Rachel Dunn-Black,** MD, owner and founder of Clarity Medical Spa, and hormone expert

"Every woman should have *Brilliant Burnout* in their library. Nisha Jackson makes an instant connection with readers because she has 'walked the talk' personally and professionally. She backs up every chapter with success stories from clients who have taken their health to the next level. Nisha understands that women are born taskmasters, and she has organized the book for the woman on the go. Each chapter stands on its own and is laid out with quizzes, research, and, most importantly, practical, insightful advice that anyone can and should put into action. This book is packed front to back with fascinating information about the mind, body, and soul. After reading this book, I am inspired to find more brilliance and to shine more luminously in my life journey."

—**Renee Sjulin,** vice president of Runza National

"Nisha Jackson has written a must-read primer that is powerful and relatable to all women of every age. *Brilliant Burnout* is inspirational, informative, and motivating and has helped me reevaluate how to balance my body, brain, and hormones while I am building my business and living a very full life with high stress.

Reading about Jackson's childhood is crucial to understanding her desire to educate women on body awareness. She explains the female hormones, and she inspires readers to feel encouraged as they experience the different stages of life—personal, business, etc. This book provides validation for all woman who want to take action in regards to their health and mind-set."

—**Nicci Jillian,** author of *Confectious Easy Desserts* and founder and owner of Confectious Pastry Shop

"I began seeing Dr. Nisha Jackson years ago, after experiencing my own burnout. Thanks to her regulating my hormones and her detailed, easy-to-follow plan for diet, exercise, and supplements, I regained my energy, vitality, and health. Most recently, I have gone through some major life changes—a divorce, relocation, a career change, and even menopause—but with Dr. Jackson's help, I not only went through this challenging chapter in my life with the strength, stamina, and clarity of thought necessary, but I also went through menopause without any of the typical negative symptoms. I am so grateful to Dr. Jackson for her expertise, care, and support. I will continue to recommend her and her book. We can feel great at any age!"

—**Linda Miner,** licensed massage therapist, health coach, functional aging specialist, and emotional freedom techniques practitioner

"Nisha Jackson has been my health practitioner for many years. My quality of life has been enhanced so much through her hormone and wellness treatments. She takes time to listen and asks questions to make the right, highly individualized plan for each patient. This is a woman's specialist who truly cares. I highly recommend Dr. Jackson to all my friends and family—she is the *best*!"

—**Charlene Phelps,** interior designer, age 56

"The quality of my life has greatly increased since I have been under Dr. Nisha Jackson's care. Her views on healthcare are totally in line with what I believe are the secrets to quality of health and aging. I am a compounding pharmacist, and I love compounding hormones. For a long time, my personal belief has been that hormones are a fountain of youth. Nisha Jackson has managed my thyroid, which has helped with my energy level and weight gain. Nisha also has balanced my progesterone, estrogen, and testosterone during menopause, which I feel helped give me a youthful enthusiasm for life. Her book very clearly spells out how to achieve balance in your own life, and I highly recommend it!"

—**Kristi Myer,** registered pharmacist, age 58

"I have known Nisha Jackson and have been a patient of hers for many years. During this time, I went through professional and personal triumphs (owning and operating 4 companies at once with over 125 employees) that caused my stress levels to reach well beyond what is normal, and my adrenal and thyroid functions were impacted to a point of total and complete exhaustion, resulting in nearly constant bed rest. Nisha Jackson saved my life. Her extensive knowledge and competent intervention, including appropriate testing, compounded hormone therapy, and medication management, turned my life around. There is no doubt in my mind that if it were not for Nisha's insight I would have likely died over 14 years ago.

Over the past several years, I have recommended her to both men and women who have shared their own success stories as well. I am pleased and proud to be one of her many patients. Reading *Brilliant Burnout* tells you how to stay at the top of your game while under tremendous pressure and stress. It will save your life if you follow the steps to stay in balance while also staying brilliant!"

—**Carolyn Souders,** PhD, BSN, LCP, RN, age 69

"Before I saw Nisha, I was mentally exhausted and lacked the energy to get daily tasks done. However, almost immediately after Nisha's complete approach at balancing my hormones, I have energy, drive, and enthusiasm and am in the best shape of my life at age 50! Her book is a must-read for every woman out there that is a 'driver' and wants to stay successful while feeling great!"

—**Dr. Randy Rothfus,** dentist and coinventor of Guzzle Buddy, age 50

"Dr. Nisha knows more about women's health than any expert I know. Her approach to hormone balance and optimization has made me a healthier and much happier person, not to mention that everyone I meet thinks I'm at least ten years younger (not easy when you're in your 60s!).

Not only is Dr. Jackson a women's health and hormone expert, but she is also a phenomenal diagnostician. I suffered from sudden onset asthma for over three years. I was treated by an expert in lung diseases and put on multiple medications. After one brief conversation with Nisha, she recognized that my exposure to fungus and mold was the likely cause. One prescription later, I was cured and forever grateful!!"

—**Linda Rogers,** PhD and laboratory scientist, age 67

"Quality of life is greatly influenced by the level of professional care we have as we age. It is just as important for men to be aware of and manage changes to our bodies as women.

Nisha helped me control my rising PSA levels with optimal levels of testosterone, which was outside of mainstream medical thinking, and now my PSA numbers are great!

I suffered a horrific near-death accident this year, breaking six ribs, five vertebrae, and my clavicle. Nisha's use of nutrient infusions, balancing all of my levels, and energetic healing, which she is trained and certified to perform, rejuvenated every cell in my body, and I got incredible results. I now feel great and have nearly fully recovered. I am boxing again, and my boxing buddies were amazed that I would even be able to get out of bed and walk, much less return to classes and exercise in 12 weeks. Nisha is truly a marvelous healer. *Brilliant Burnout* is a must-read for any woman wanting to stay in the game long-term. Staying balanced the way that Nisha spells out in her book is an absolute necessity for long-term success without falling prey to fatigue, depression, and accelerated aging."

—**Robert Meyer,** serial entrepreneur, age 71

"As a mental health therapist working with women of all ages, I wholeheartedly agree with Dr. Jackson's holistic approach to health and wellness. Today, it is more common to prescribe an antidepressant than to look at the root of the problem, which can often be remedied by hormone replacement, diet changes, self-care, and making lifestyle changes.

This book is a practical guide for women asking the question, 'Can I have it all?' We need to learn to balance our busy lives, deciding what our priorities are and what no longer serves us. When I first became a patient of Dr. Jackson, I was experiencing symptoms of stress, anxiety, fatigue, lack of focus, low sex drive, and sleep problems. After making changes in my diet, taking supplements, and using hormone pellet therapy, my symptoms decreased significantly. Almost immediately, I noticed improvements in my physical, mental, and emotional health and well-being. It has truly been life changing!"

—**Angela Fogg,** MA and NCC, age 54

"My experience with Dr. Nisha and the staff at Peak Medical Clinic have far exceeded my expectations. It has been a life-changing experience! After having had a hysterectomy at a young age, I had been unknowingly suffering the exhausting effects of hormonal imbalance. Having an established, successful, and busy career as a nanny left no time for unexplained exhaustion. By luck, a girlfriend told me about a book Dr. Nisha Jackson had written. Reading it was a game changer for me. I now do not know what I would have done without this book! My next step was to go meet with Dr. Nisha Jackson.

After receiving my results, Nisha gave me a plan to put me on track with my hormones, diet, supplements and the perfect plan for lifestyle changes and stress management. Within a few days of returning home and going back to work, my exhaustion was gone!

My friends keep telling me 'You look great, your attitude is so positive, and where did you get all this energy?'"

—**Kathy Hunter,** executive nanny, age 41

"I have always said, the world needs more women like Nisha, but God only made one! *Brilliant Burnout* is more than encouragement; it's a road map for women to drive away from burnout."

—**Jason Atkinson,** film producer, American politician, and international lecturer

"Dr. Nisha Jackson is the living embodiment of what she's written about! I've known Nisha for over 20 years. She's a leader in the wellness and healthy aging market. Her positive outlook, backed by a scientific approach, encourages women of all ages to be their best selves. Writing this book is one more way for Nisha to continue her mission to support women in their life-long journey toward health and happiness."

—**Shelley Thode,** CEO of SLIM/PROtherapies, Inc.

"Nisha pays attention to the fine details of her patient's needs. She is confident and patient and gives you 100 percent of her attention while in her presence. Nisha is ahead of the curve in the fields of hormone replacement therapy and total body balance and wellness. She has been my 'Balance Doc' for over 20 years."

—**Kim Nelson,** realtor, massage therapist,
and healthcare advocate, age 51

"I have had the absolute honor and privilege to have Nisha as my doctor for over 20 years. I am 67, and at age 45 was going through menopause. My estrogen levels had tanked, and I was very emotional and constantly on the verge of tears. With persistence, diligence, and hormone therapy, over a few months she got me straightened out. She not only cares about my healthcare but cares about me as a person. I have never felt like just a number, and I consider her a warmhearted, caring friend!"

—**Debbie Dauenhauer,** age 67

"Ladies, buy this book. Your health matters. You can't pour from an empty cup, and *Brilliant Burnout* will give you what you need to fill it up!

Nisha has written this book for each one of us. She writes from a place of personal experience and is raw, honest, and SO relatable. *Brilliant Burnout* will give you the tools to make smarter decisions about your own health and the ability to put it all together. This is a must-read for any woman who is trying to live her best life but finds herself hitting the wall, day in and day out."

—**Shannon Cronin,** age 46

"As a woman in my late 20s driven to accomplish it *all*—career, relationships, and happiness—sometimes I relate burnout to weakness. When, in fact, I am my biggest asset. Taking care of my body and being mindful is so important, and Nisha's tips are life changing. This is a must-read!"

—**Maddy Brown,** New York Jets Community Relations, age 26

BRILLIANT BURNOUT

HOW SUCCESSFUL, DRIVEN WOMEN
CAN STAY IN THE GAME BY REWIRING THEIR
BODIES, BRAINS, AND HORMONES

NISHA JACKSON, PhD, MS, NP, HHP

RIVER GROVE
BOOKS

This book is intended as a reference volume only, not as a medical manual. The information given here is designed to help you make informed decisions about your health. It is not intended as a substitute for any treatment that may have been prescribed by your doctor. If you suspect that you have a medical problem, you should seek competent medical help. You should not begin a new health regimen without first consulting a medical professional.

Published by River Grove Books
Austin, TX
www.rivergrovebooks.com

Distributed by River Grove Books

Design and composition by Greenleaf Book Group and Kim Lance
Cover design by Greenleaf Book Group and Kim Lance

Publisher's Cataloging-in-Publication data is available.

Print ISBN: 978-1-63299-210-9

eBook ISBN: 978-1-63299-211-6

First Edition

This book is dedicated to my grandmother—my Nana, Jessie.

She is a brilliant firecracker, a role model, and the most amazing lady I know. At 98 years old, she continues to be full of life. She's a strong, independent woman. She lives alone and even still drives herself any-place she wants to go. She is completely engaged in life and giving back, and she takes care of everyone around her. Jessie has survived more hardships and trials than any one person should endure, but she still gets up every morning, eats a perfectly balanced diet, reads, moves her body (despite the aches and pains), stays connected socially, takes her supple-ments (she's still on hormones, for heaven's sake), and always takes time for those she loves. She is the best example of how to live your life to the fullest. She takes care of herself and makes every moment count. I love you more than I could ever say, Nana. XO.

Contents

Introduction

bril•liant

/ˈbril-yənt/

1. (of light or color) very bright and radiant.
synonyms: bright, shining, dazzling, intense, gleaming, luminous, radiant

2. exceptionally clever or talented.
synonyms: bright, intelligent, clever, smart, astute, intellectual

THIS DEFINITION OF *brilliant* is the one that you are likely to find in any dictionary or web search. It's succinct, clear, and boring. But it is also incomplete. To me, the word *brilliant* is not only about being smart or insightful; it's also a state of being that falls more closely in line with the first definition, where a person's inner light shines brightly on the world around them.

When I call a person brilliant, I'm saying that they are kind, hardworking, loving, tenacious, charitable, determined, nurturing, healthy, fun, and yes, even smart. I'm saying that their life has a positive effect on the world and people around them. It is the highest compliment I can give. This is the definition of brilliant I want you to carry in your mind as you read through this book, because it's the one I am using. For much of my life, people have called me brilliant, but it took a long time before I was capable of thinking that way of myself, and now I have dedicated my life to helping other people realize their unique brilliance.

For women in the modern world, finding and maintaining our brilliance has gotten harder than ever. We want to work, have families, make a difference, fall in love, be leaders, and still be strong, beautiful, and healthy women—but the odds seem to always be stacked against us. And when you are determined and unwilling to accept defeat, as many of us are, the stress of attaining these goals can literally begin to kill us. This state is called *burnout*, and it's something many women are intimately familiar with.

That's where this book comes in. I want to teach you how to optimize your health, relationships, and mental fortitude so you can let your brilliant self shine its absolute brightest. But why, you might be asking, should you take my advice? The simple answer is because I've been in your shoes. I have spent my entire life researching and falling victim to burnout, and now I am finally at a point where I can share what I've learned to help other women defeat stress and start living their best lives. The longer answer requires me to go back in time a bit, so you can understand where I'm coming from.

A CONFESSION

I'm going to start my story with a confession. I'm a workaholic. It's true; I always have been. As insane as this may sound, when I turned nine, I asked my father for the chance to work in his A&W restaurant for the day. My father, an entrepreneur, felt this would be a good opportunity for me to learn the value of hard work, so he agreed. I was told to stand on a five-gallon pickle bucket (so I could see into the dining room) and watch for customers to finish their meals and leave. Then I would dart out, grab their trays, and enthusiastically clean the tabletops. That day, I got a taste of the hard work that would become an addiction, catapulting me into a lifetime of workaholism. But I needed to do more than bus tables to get my "fix." From there, I started creating things—little things like macramé hangers, découpage, and toile paintings—and found local stores where I could sell these little jewels around town. I eventually turned my tiny walk-in closet into my shop, where I spent a ridiculous amount of time making my little creations. I couldn't get enough of work, and what's more, I found out that I really liked making money. I certainly wasn't your typical nine-year-old. (I don't think my parents knew what to do with me.)

I began really working at age 11, both at my parent's restaurants and in department stores, putting together mannequins' outfits and selling clothes. When I wasn't at either of my jobs, I would follow my mother and grandmother around, learning how to cook and clean, and by the age of 12, I could easily cook or bake nearly anything.

My father was a business owner, and I learned so much from him as well. Every night, I would help cook dinner, and then my father would come home and sit at the dinner table, ranting about employee or work problems as we ate. I hung on every word he said because I knew he was right.

I stayed focused on my jobs throughout junior high and high school. However, as I neared the end of my high school years, I came to a crossroads. Suddenly, I realized I had no idea what I was going to do with my life—my family had never talked about college because my parents and most of my family had not pursued education any further than a high school diploma. I was at a loss for what to do next. I had all the passion and work ethic I needed, and I wanted to do so many things, but I had little to no guidance on what career I should pursue, other than I should have a job and make money, and I wasn't sure where I should focus my energy.

FINDING PURPOSE

A real turning point in my life came when I spent the summer after my junior year of high school traveling around China with a group of kids from the United States. During this trip, I came down with a bad case of dysentery and spent a few days in a hospital in Shanghai. It had dirt floors, and their methods of healing weren't what I was used to—it was as if I had traveled back in time. I watched as the Chinese doctors who worked on me used techniques of acupuncture, application of herbal balms, tincture pellets, and oils, taking me from deathly ill to better than ever in less than 48 hours. It was a miraculous transformation, and this experience stuck with me.

I was captivated by how the Chinese used so many different modalities that I had never seen or heard of to heal me. It was like a coordinated attack on what was making me sick. I returned home from that trip and knew that I wanted to go into medicine. I wanted to make a difference and to try to understand the true nature of healing.

After I graduated high school, I went to college, got my bachelor's degree in nursing, and became an RN. I married my college sweetheart and moved from Southern California to Southern Oregon. It was a happy time in my life, but it wasn't long before I realized I needed more out of my career. I wanted to be in charge, to make decisions, and to be more involved in my patients' care. Besides, I wasn't working nearly hard enough yet. So, I took a chance and made a *big* change. I launched myself into a master's program, followed by an OB/GYN nurse practitioner program and a PhD program. I could feel myself getting closer to what I was truly meant to do—working with and helping women.

A WOMAN'S TOUCH

After I got my degree and became a nurse practitioner in a private OB/GYN practice, it wasn't long before my world was rocked yet again. One of my first patients told me she had been on various hormones for menopause and yet she still had hot flashes and night sweats. She also suffered from exhaustion, was gaining weight, and had no sex drive. I noticed she had tried various forms of hormone therapy (all pharmaceuticals), and none of them seemed to make any difference at all. There was no other formal treatment method at that time, so I had to admit that I had no other options for her. I will never forget her looking at me and saying, "Is this it? Is this all you can offer?"

I couldn't get her words out of my head, and I knew she wasn't alone. I wondered how many other women were experiencing the same frustrations. I went back to my office and sat there thinking, *There must be more we can do for these women who still feel terrible on the standard hormone therapy. Why hasn't someone figured this out?* I decided right then and there to take on the task myself.

Thus began the greatest intellectual journey of my life. I learned about diet, hormone testing, the use of bioidentical hormones, supplementation, nonstandard medicine modalities, acupuncture, mind-body therapies, herbal treatments, and anything else I could find that might improve a women's emotional, mental, and physical state of being as she aged. I spent thousands of hours reading, asking questions, training with outside specialists, and attending conferences. I was that weird girl at work who was always reading books during the lunch hour and starting conversations about ovaries (which, to be honest, is not that weird in an OB/GYN office).

As I put the pieces of the puzzle together, all my research started to pay off because I realized I could actually help these women. And the more I learned, the more I realized that I liked the work. In fact, I couldn't get enough of it. I started some of my patients on new diets; tested their hormones and worked to balance levels that were out of the ideal range; and implemented herbs, vitamins, and minerals for specific ailments. And guess what… my patients began transforming before my eyes. Women began feeling better, losing weight, sleeping better, having great sex, and, of course, telling their closest friends all about their progress. The word about my work and what I was doing spread, and I couldn't have been happier.

Soon after I saw that the treatments were working, I put together a pilot program for aging women, which included a full financial pro forma to present to the all-male board of directors at the large multispecialty group where I worked. You can probably already guess where this is going... Within the first 20 minutes of my presentation, they interrupted me and told me that, despite all my evidence, they were not interested in any type of "complementary medicine" helping women age more slowly, or even embarking on anything that deviated from the USRDA food pyramid (6–11 bread servings a day—yikes!). The board thought it was a bad idea, so they unanimously voted it down. But I wasn't going to let them stop me. The next day, I gave my notice and left the practice to go out on my own. I was the first nurse practitioner in Southern Oregon to open her own private practice. Take that, patriarchy! My brilliant journey was just beginning.

MORE BALLS IN THE AIR

Unfortunately, success with my clients did not mean my life was getting any easier. By this time, I had two daughters and had built two homes. After I opened my own practice and gave birth to my youngest daughter, Kenzie, I realized I was burning the proverbial candle at both ends. I felt guilty whenever I spent more time with the girls than at the office or vice versa. I was sick, tired, foggy, depressed, and irritable, and I couldn't sleep. I was feeling burned out, but I didn't know that was my condition at the time. I was all in on the new adventure of starting my own practice and knew in my heart that it was the right thing to do for my career and for all the women out there, but I also felt run down—physically, mentally, and emotionally.

WHOLE-BODY REBOOT

I finally realized that it was time to practice what I preached. I needed a whole-body reboot—STAT! I tested my hormones and found that I had rock-bottom progesterone (mood hormone) levels, a low thyroid level, and Hashimoto's thyroiditis. It wasn't good news, but now that I knew what was wrong, I could figure out my battle plan. I began a new routine of sleeping better and eating a low-sugar diet. I also implemented herbs and B-12 shots, and I treated my tired adrenal glands and optimized my thyroid with medication. It was—cue the hallelujah chorus—a miracle. I instantly felt better, and the way I was handling my work and children improved too. What's more, I knew for sure that the system I was prescribing my patients worked. So, I plunged forward.

My new practice was booming, and before long I was hiring additional medical providers, but I needed to work overtime to get them trained. As my business grew, I had to develop new treatment programs while still seeing patients, taking care of my kids, and trying to stay balanced. In the midst of all this, my husband had a change in career, and circumstances became even more difficult. And what do we hardworking women do when things get difficult? Self-care. Just kidding. We buckle down and work three times harder.

I took on another practice, agreeing to help design a new space and become the managing partner of a large OB/GYN clinic, while still growing my own practice. I began a nutraceutical company, Balance Docs, which formulated supplements that were the highest quality and dosage for optimal effects, and a clinical laboratory business, Rogue Clinical Labs, so we could have the most accurate lab results for our patients in a controlled environment. I told myself all this extra stress was okay because, after all, I was healthy now. But inside, my resolve was starting to crumble.

BURNOUT 2.0

For the second time in only a few short years, I had pushed myself too far, and I couldn't even blame it on my hormones this time. I was creating new businesses and filling needs in the field of functional medicine that I knew needed to be filled. At the same time, I wanted to continue to see my patients, and I found myself having trouble saying no. I was immersed in my work, which I enjoyed, and I didn't want to compromise, but I knew that I had to do something to take care of myself.

I began to realize that the spiritual part of myself was neglected, so I read every book about mind-body relaxation and meditation that I could get my hands on. I attended conferences and trainings and underwent hundreds of personal treatments. I had spent every ounce of my energy taking care of everything and everyone else in my life. I had nothing left for me.

I could also see that this burnout was a common thread for highly energetic, successful women. And, obviously, when we give everything we have away and have nothing left for ourselves, the consequences can be dire. So I did the same thing I now recommend to all my patients who come in with burnout: I started meditating and paying attention to what I truly wanted in my life. I began riding my horse more, spending more time with friends, and reaching out for help when I needed it (which was hard for me).

After implementing these changes, I felt a renewed sense of purpose and decided to foster my creative side. Of course, I'm not the kind of gal who does anything small. So, in addition to my full-time (and then some) career, I began designing homes and working in the real-estate market. By the time our girls were in junior high, my husband and I had purchased 15 homes, remodeled or rebuilt them, designed and decorated the interiors, and rented or even lived in them ourselves. We moved about every two to four years. While this may sound crazy, it was actually great fun and a wonderful source of added revenue. After awhile, however, this lifestyle took its toll on me, because, *of course*, it would.

NEXT-LEVEL BURNOUT

In 2010, I hit another wall. My integrative medicine clinic had grown to be a large operation with more than 70 employees, including medical doctors, nurse practitioners, chiropractors, acupuncturists, and nutritionists. In addition, we had two busy, athletic daughters, 4 horses, 13 chickens, 4 dogs, 2 cats, 20 acres, a vineyard, and I was starting to design, develop, and build a winery and tasting room on our property (because, really, what's the point of having a vineyard otherwise, right?). Just when my life could not get any crazier, I again reached a point where I simply couldn't do it anymore. As wonderful as everything was, as blessed and privileged as I had been, I had grown to *hate* my life. This was when I hit next-level burnout.

Ultimately, I had been fooling myself all along. I thought that since I was taking excellent care of myself by exercising faithfully, eating well, taking supplements, balancing my hormones, and being vigilant about sleeping eight hours every night, that it would be okay to continue piling things on. It turns out, I lacked major boundaries in my work life. I was so immersed in my work that it was defining me, and, as a result, I found myself not liking who I had become.

Once again, I had to swallow my pride and take my own advice. I had no choice but to make changes in my home life and ask for help. I sold my interest in the OB/GYN practice and the integrative medicine clinic after 21 years of owning and managing them. In their place, I opened a more boutique-style functional medicine practice, Peak Medical, with a focus on slowing the aging process for men and women. (I just had to do something; I told you that I'm a workaholic.) This time, however, I made sure not to overextend myself by keeping the practice focused and simple (and, of course, brilliant).

Peak Medical is now in its third year of business and is strategically expanding to other cities throughout the Northwest, only this time I'm managing the growth of my business in a saner fashion, surrounded by people I love and trust wholeheartedly. It took me a while, but I think I may have finally figured out how to be a hardworking, brilliant woman without literally killing myself.

FINALLY FIGURING THINGS OUT

What I have learned through this lifelong process of being a driven, passionate, entrepreneurial junkie in search of my own brilliance is that there is only one way to achieve whole-body wellness: *balance*. You must have balance in all areas of your life. You will never be able to keep all the balls in the air if you are not doing what you need to do to take care of *yourself* first. I have treated and counseled thousands of patients in my career, most of whom I have had tremendous success with, but nothing compares to my own firsthand experience. After many years of hard work and being extremely successful and yet simultaneously scraping the bottom of the burnout barrel, I get it. If you are reading this book because you are on the edge of burnout or fully immersed in the trenches of stress, I want you to know first and foremost that I understand what you are going through.

At age 55, I have had more brilliant burnouts than I'd like to admit. While they have been, in every sense of the word, true burnouts, I like to refer to them as necessary turning points in my life. Not because it's any more true. It just sounds better. But let me be clear: I didn't write this book because I needed another project. I wrote it for the brilliant women out there who are making a difference in the world by raising children, managing their careers, starting businesses, creating amazing things, and running companies. I have a burning desire to support these women in their own quest for success and to educate and coach them on how to navigate their way through life in the healthiest and most balanced fashion. We need brilliant women in the world now more than ever, and it is my mission to get them the energy they need to stay in the game.

The most amazing thing about brilliant women, though, is how we are able to teach and support each other along the way. I set out to write this book to help other women find balance in their own health, in the midst of total chaos, using my personal and clinical experience. But as I began writing about my own reflections and experiences, reaching out to past patients and female colleagues and doing more research into the clinical evidence of the methods we have consistently used in our medical practice, something amazing happened. I ended up finding even more balance and peace within myself along the way. I changed, modified, and removed things from my life that were tripping me up and keeping me off center to make more room for the lovely things that I need more of to stay balanced. Writing this book has honestly been one of the greatest privileges, and I can't wait for you to use it to start making your life even more brilliant than it already is.

HOW TO USE THIS BOOK

One thing I know about brilliant women is they know how to get things done, regardless of how full their lives are. And this book is designed for busy women. You can read it from cover to cover or use it to help with specific issues that are creating burnout in your life right now. If you are experiencing next-level burnout, then, frankly, you've got no time to waste. Scan the table of contents, see which issue speaks loudest to you, and go directly to that chapter. No judgment here. Promise.

Each chapter begins with a quiz to help you gauge how pressing that specific issue is in your life at that moment. And each chapter ends with a series of tips to help you get on the fast track to feeling better. Again, though, I know you're busy. And if reading an entire chapter seems too daunting right now, try simply taking the chapter quiz, reading the tips, and beginning the fast-track plan at the end of the chapter. I just want you to get started.

I worked hard to make sure this book works for you, no matter your schedule or reading habits. The chapters are meant to give you more energy, stamina, strength, balance, sex drive (ooh-la-la), mental performance, mood boosts, weight loss, and antiaging effects—and are meant to be quickly and easily implemented into what is surely an already overloaded schedule.

Most importantly, I want this book to offer you hope. If you feel as though your life is over or that you will never have the energy, good mood, brain function, and drive for success you once had, then I am here to tell you that you are *wrong*. You can. If you are ready to make some simple, highly effective changes to take your health to the next level, while improving your own brilliant mind, then this book is for you. It will be an excellent guide for you both personally and professionally; you just need to turn the page…

I wish you the best in your journey with your own unique brilliance. You deserve every ounce of it!

Nisha Jackson, PhD, MS, NP, HHP

1

Today's Classic Burnout: Having It All . . . Including the Stress

"Find your balance and stand with it. Find your song and sing it out. Find your cadence and let it appear like a dance. Find the questions that only you know how to ask and the answers that you are content to not know."

—MARY ANNE RADMACHER

IN THIS CHAPTER, we're going to be discussing burnout and how it can affect women, both mentally and physically. To see where you fall on the burnout spectrum, take a moment to answer the following quiz.

QUIZ: ARE YOU BURNED OUT?

Answer the following questions as honestly as you can, based on how you feel now. After you've completed the quiz, add up your total number of "yes" answers.

1. No matter how much sleep you get, do you wake up feeling tired and unrested? Y/N

2. Do you hit a wall in the afternoon? Y/N

3. Do you have sugar, salt, or starch cravings that you can't seem to get under control? Y/N

4. Are you using alcohol, food, or drugs in the evening or after work to relax? Y/N

5. Do you need to use something to increase energy throughout the day, such as caffeine, prescribed medicines, or supplements? Y/N

6. Are you easily irritated by small problems or by coworkers or family? Y/N

7. Do you have negative thoughts about your job and feel you are not getting out what you are putting into it? Y/N

8. Do you feel unsupported by your spouse or feel you are doing the majority of the work in your household? Y/N

9. Do you often experience unexplained sadness? Y/N

10. Are you forgetting appointments or deadlines, or are you losing personal possessions (like your keys) regularly? Y/N

11. Are you seeing family members and friends less frequently? Y/N

12. Are you too busy to make routine phone calls, read reports, or remember birthdays or celebrations? Y/N

13. Are you unable to laugh at a joke about yourself? Y/N

14. Does sex seem like more trouble than its worth? Y/N

15. Are you experiencing more PMS or menopausal or hormonal changes? Y/N

16. Do you gain weight easily, especially around the belly? Y/N

17. Do you feel your skin is aging or feel as if you're aging too quickly? Y/N

18. Are you experiencing anxiety or does your heart race often? Y/N

19. Are you experiencing increased physical complaints (body pain, headaches, lingering colds or flu)? Y/N

20. Do you have brain fog and lack of focus and memory? Y/N

21. Do you feel you are achieving less than you should? Y/N

Total number of yes answers: _____

1–5 yes answers: You might be okay for now, but be careful because you are at risk of burning out. Now is the best time to implement new strategies to achieve balance.

6–10 yes answers: You can't keep doing this to yourself; you've got moderate burnout. It is time to change at least three areas of your life to adjust your course.

11–15 yes answers: Danger! We've got work to do. You are suffering from significant burnout. You should make diet, sleep, and hormone changes in the next 90 days.

16–21 yes answers: You might want to sit down for this—you've got severe burnout. This should be treated immediately through diet, hormone adjustments, brain support, lifestyle adjustments, and supplementation.

After completing this quiz, you should have a good idea of where you are on the burnout scale. And no matter how severe your burnout is, the good news is that you are close to discovering real solutions to overcoming this state.

ON THE EDGE OF BURNOUT

Today, most women are constantly dealing with an undercurrent of stress in their lives. We all have it rough in this day and age, but studies show that women have twice the level of stress and stress-related disorders (such as anxiety, depression, and physical problems tied to stress) as men do.[1]

In fact, numerous studies have shown that high-achieving women have a constant internal turmoil that is detrimental to their health and quality of life.[2] This is something that I find simply unacceptable. More than that, I consider burnout for these brilliant women a tragedy. High-achieving, driven, passionate women everywhere are maxed out, addicted to being busy, and thriving on chaos (or at least fooling themselves into thinking that they're thriving). Keeping busy at all costs is now the cultural norm, but, if brilliant women took a moment to realistically consider what they were doing to themselves, they might take a step back and start taking on less. Manic busyness can lead to

- Exhaustion

- Guilt

- Anxiety

- Social comparison (a cousin of FOMO, or fear of missing out)

- Inauthenticity

- Significant physical and mental symptoms

The inner drive to do more and achieve more is significantly impacting women's health, families, and careers. And one of the problems with

---

1   M. Pilar Matud, "Gender Differences in Stress and Coping Styles," *Science Direct* 37, no. 7 (2004): 1401–1415, doi: 10.1016/j. paid.2004.01.010.

2   "Americans Engage in Unhealthy Behaviors to Manage Stress," American Psychological Association, February 23, 2006, https://www.apa.org/news/press/releases/2006/01/stress-management.aspx.

burnout is that it's so intricately woven into women's lives that even the brightest of women are not able to identify the telltale signs until it is too late. The path to burnout is caused by a complex and interacting web of stressors, but they all boil down to a few key causes:

- Women's expanded roles (home, career, children, parents)

- Constant sensory stimulation

- Social pressures to achieve more and have more

- Family and child expectations

- Financial constraints

- Poor lifestyle habits (sleep, diet, exercise, hormone imbalances, and brain chemical deficiencies)

- Adrenaline addiction

You must also remember that getting burned out is not your fault, because it simply isn't. It's something that has insidiously made its way into the constructs of modern society and become the norm. These days, women are expected to take on more than they can handle, so burnout has become more common. The brilliant woman may be able to sustain the chaos for some time, but the stress will eventually take its toll. Full-throttle burnout can take months or years to manifest, but a meltdown is inevitable.

Over the past 25 years, but primarily in the past five years, I have witnessed significant burnout in colleagues, friends, family, and thousands of patients. I have seen countless women who once had sparkles in their eyes and fires in their bellies–driving them toward adventure, challenge, and pursuing their passions–eventually fall victim to intense fatigue, depression, anxiety, health decline, and loss of zest for life. Their flame simply went out.

Burnout is a villain that quietly and skillfully robs women of what makes them brilliant, and it's effective because of its gradual onset that works below the surface, traveling methodically through each of its stages, ultimately leaving women feeling lost and desperate, with no clue how they got there or what to do about it. If you feel constantly rushed or in a hurry and can't seem to catch up, but you still want more from your life and know you are too young and too smart to jump ship, then I am here to tell you that you are not alone.

To help you avoid getting to this state, it's important to be aware of the triggers of burnout so you can understand how it sneaks into our lives so easily. Can you recognize any of the following triggers in your own life?

TRIGGERS FOR BURNOUT

- **Interrupted sleep or insomnia:** This can manifest in anxiety, fatigue, and a lack of focus.
- **Poor diet:** This can lead to a disturbance in brain chemicals, which causes irritability, cravings, and depression.
- **Intense pressure on self:** This happens when you push yourself too far. This can lead to a drop in progesterone, causing mood instability, PMS, early menopausal symptoms, and irregular cycles; it can even stop ovulation.
- **Lack of movement or exercise:** This can result in shortened temper, anxiety, pent-up stress (no outlet), weight gain, body pain, and a loss of flexibility and strength.
- **Eating foods high in sugar or bad carbs and snacking and skipping**

meals that contain protein, good carbs, and fat: More than just having a poor diet, these eating habits specifically cause higher insulin levels or low or unstable blood sugar levels that result in weight gain, an inability to concentrate, headaches, and memory loss.

- **Shallow breathing:** When you fail to take in deeper breaths, you are sending a signal to your body that you are in fight-or-flight mode. This can cause headaches, fuzzy brain, unstable cortisol levels, and a constant state of activation (a medical term for overstimulation).

- **Hypertasking:** Moving quickly and unconsciously between tasks with interruptions creates an inability to stay focused. You can also lose personal items, forget appointments, and experience confusion, dizziness, and rage.

- **Saying yes to one more thing:** Overextending yourself can lead to anger, poor execution of tasks, resentment, a cynical attitude, and a negative state of mind.

- **Limited social connections:** This can lead to more anger and pent-up frustration. A lack of connection negatively affects the adrenal stress system, leading to a downward spiral.

- **Limited alone time:** When you have no time to step back and examine what is happening in your life and what you can do about it, you end up reaching a boiling point with symptoms of irritability and the emotional exaggeration of stress (i.e., rage, irrational behavior, and making decisions that are not in your best interest due to not getting the right perspective or having the right priorities).

- **Lack of necessary supplementation, hormone testing, and age or stress intervention:** This can cause an imbalance in the endocrine system, often stemming from overworked, underperforming adrenal glands.

- **No time for planning:** Poor use of time leads to bad food choices, lack of sleep, and increased stress—emotionally, mentally, and physically.

It is easy to see how these triggers can make their way into your life. There are a limited number of hours in the day, and trying to keep yourself healthy by planning ahead, eating regularly, slowing down a few hours before you go to bed to shift your body into sleep mode, keeping yourself tuned up with supplements and hormones, and turning off your brain when it gets away from you takes more than simply a burning desire to feel better. It takes practice, commitment, and an extreme devotion to self-care.

THE 12 STAGES OF BURNOUT

If you are like me, you may find yourself annoyed at the advice "Just relax and slow down" or "Just let it go" or "Stop worrying about everything so much." (My eye started to twitch just writing that.) I have never been knee-deep in seven different projects and thought, *If I just let it go and relax, everything will be okay.* That simply isn't part of my DNA. Instead, I tend to be a bit bullheaded about things; I am more action oriented and results driven. I still choose to believe that women *can* have it all, but now I recognize that they need to go about getting it the right way (which, of course, is going to require some letting go of worry and relaxing).

Today, you and other brilliant women's long-term success is based on a commitment to strategically managing yourself in all areas of your life. Doing this requires that you preserve your brain, empower your adrenals, keep fit and healthy, and be able to withstand daily stressors and stay on top of things while feeling optimally balanced.

There are various stages of burnout that I have researched extensively in my efforts to fight it. To keep it simple, I will briefly outline them here. This list will show you how burnout progresses. And in the figure, you will see how your body responds to the stress of burnout.

The Body's Response to HIGH STRESS

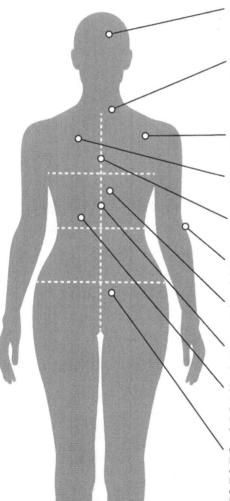

HEAD
Issues with mood, anger, confusion, memory loss, lack of concentration, anxiety, depression, cravings, addictions, state of nervous system activation—sympathetic

THYROID
Lower thyroid production, compromised conversion of T4 (storage) to T3 (active) thyroid, fatigue, weight gain, dry skin, puffy eyes, memory and mood decline, cracking heels and elbows, skin problems, digestion problems, inflammation, high cholesterol

SKIN
Acne, psoriasis, eczema, dermatitis, random breakouts, skin rashes

LUNGS
Rapid shallow breathing leading to headaches, anxiety, shortness of breath, dizziness, light-headed

HEART
Racing heart, palpitations, high blood pressure, increased risk of heart attack and stroke

JOINTS AND MUSCLES
Aches and pains, inflammation, tension, reduced bone density, tightness in shoulders and back

ADRENALS
Inflammation, weight gain, nervous, irritable, allergies, hypersensitivities to foods, exhaustion, body pain

IMMUNE SYSTEM (PANCREAS)
Recurrent illness, sickness, flu/viruses, susceptible to autoimmune disorders

STOMACH/PANCREAS/LIVER
Irritable bowel, diarrhea, constipation, poor absorption of nutrients, reduced metabolism, candida, heart burn, reflux, nausea, cramping, skin tags, elevated insulin, diabetes and obesity

OVARIES
Lack of ovulation, low progesterone, testosterone and estradiol- infertility, low sex drive, heavy periods, irregular bleeding, sore breasts, cystic breasts and ovaries, hot flashes, night sweats, insomnia, fatigue, PMS, early menopausal symptoms

Figure 1.1: The Body's Response to High Stress

12 STAGES OF BURNOUT

....

- Stage 1: **Burning desire.** This happens when your inner drive to work hard and get ahead while proving yourself kicks in.
- Stage 2: **Intense working.** This is when you establish high personal goals (many times unrealistic in scope), often with a myopic focus on work while family, home, and friends get moved to the back burner.
- Stage 3: **Starting to ignore personal needs.** This happens when your personal needs (such as the importance of good sleep, exercise, supplementation, and regular meals) begin to be ignored.
- Stage 4: **Personal neglect.** After a period of ignoring your personal needs, you eventually reach a state of personal neglect. At this stage, you notice health issues (such as gaining weight, not sleeping well, and eating junk food). While knowing you are not at your best, you continue to postpone getting back on track to a later date, "when things calm down."
- Stage 5: **Displacement of priorities.** This is when your work consumes all your energy, leaving little for family and friends. You also start feeling overworked and underappreciated at this stage.
- Stage 6: **Onset of physical and emotional problems related to stress.** Here you begin to experience: fatigue during the day; headaches; flying off the handle at those you love; and forgetting obviously important dates, names, and details that begin affecting your production at work, your homelife, and your ultimate success. At this stage, you might find yourself thinking, *I've lost my mind. What is wrong with me?*
- Stage 7: **Withdrawal.** This occurs over time, but true withdrawal happens when you find yourself saying, "I just don't want to see anyone" and have minimal social contact. This behavior is often coupled with the use, or abuse, of alcohol or drugs to take the edge off.
- Stage 8: **Behavioral changes.** At this stage, others are telling you that they are worried about you and your stress level, and you become aware that

you are overreacting to normal day-to-day issues or problems that arise (e.g., your kids don't pick up their room and you go postal).

- Stage 9: **Loss of drive.** This is when you begin to no longer see yourself as useful; you feel you have lost your edge and no longer have the drive you used to have. This is the stage where you begin to think about quitting your job, sending your kids to grandma's, leaving your partner, and heading to Mexico in a stolen Porsche. This stage is also known as "You are desperate and feel you have no other options."

- Stage 10: **Inner emptiness.** At this stage, you have little to no enthusiasm for work, home, or others. You begin engaging in destructive habits to overcome these feelings (such as asking your medical provider for medications to wake up, to sleep, to help your mood, anxiety, and focus, which all have their own side effects). Often at this stage, you exhibit increasing use of alcohol and drugs and spontaneous destructive behavior.

- Stage 11: **Depression.** This progresses over time, but by the time you notice it, you are already deep in its throes. When you reach this stage, you feel true exhaustion, depression, anxiety, and hopelessness and may even be questioning your life, mission, and value.

- Stage 12: **Burnout.** By the time you reach this stage, you can no longer connect with work or family and find yourself collapsing physically, mentally, and emotionally. This is the brilliant woman's rock bottom.

. . . .

Burnout can negatively affect every part of your body. That's the bad news. *But* there's some good news, too. You have control over every single activity that can help you recover, and I'm going to show you how.

THE ENDOCRINE TRIAD STRESS SYSTEM

To grasp the concept of how your body reacts to stress and how it protects you, let's take a quick look at the endocrine system.

On the offensive line for stress are three endocrine glands: the ovaries, adrenals, and thyroid. These three glands work together and are inseparable. Also included in the stress management system for women are neurochemicals in the brain, the gastrointestinal system, nervous system, and, of course, the human psyche, or will.

When your body is under stress, high levels of stress-modulating hormones and neurotransmitters (such as cortisol, norepinephrine, epinephrine, dopamine, and serotonin) are released. This is a natural and healthy response to a stressful situation. Once the event passes, your body returns to a state of non-stress, and your hormone and neurotransmitter levels decline. However, if you're dealing with continuous stress, your body will not be able to return to a relaxed, non-stressed state. Instead, you will continue to produce stress-regulating hormones and neurotransmitters to assist with the constant movement between one event and the next. You can probably guess by now where this leads…

"But is stress really that big of a deal?" People ask me this all the time. "An emotional breakdown isn't going to kill me," they say. And ignoring the fact that they're wrong about that for now, I like to point out that stress has more than just emotional effects. If you've been exposed to continuous high levels of stress hormones, chemicals, and neurotransmitters, over time, your body will move into a state of malfunction, adversely affecting your endocrine system, brain, nervous system, and metabolism. This, in turn, causes your hormones and transmitters to become depleted, resulting in numerous detrimental and unwanted symptoms.

There are serious physical consequences of unattended, ill-managed stress. Adrenal hypofunction, neurotransmitter imbalances, and ovarian hormone dysregulation are all consequences of unchecked stress. Each one of these dysfunctions leads to a list of unwanted symptoms, such as depression, anxiety, memory loss, insomnia, headaches, tachycardia (racing heart), food cravings, hypoglycemia (low blood sugar), allergies, hypersensitivities, an inability to manage stress emotionally, excessive storage of fat, type 2 diabetes, and even addictions.

It's important to know about the endocrine system and the many ways it can affect our wellness. The entire endocrine system is interconnected and always seeking optimal balance, so when we have a problem with burnout, we need to address the entire system. Let's look at some of the key players in our endocrine system and how they are affected by stress.

Cortisol

Cortisol, the primary hormone called upon for stress, is something you have probably heard of before; it tends to get a bad rap. But the truth is that it is necessary in optimal levels to be able to manage your stress, both physically and mentally. When cortisol becomes too low, it becomes difficult to navigate through stressful situations without losing it, having a breakdown, or finding yourself exhausted and overly emotional.

The Adrenal Glands

The adrenal glands, along with the hypothalamus and pituitary gland, are one of the main systems involved in coping with stress. If they are not functioning adequately, your ability to react normally to stress is lost. Adrenal hypofunction or fatigue occurs when your adrenal glands become exhausted from too much stress and they no longer perform their functions as required. They've essentially become desensitized. This can lead to problems with insulin-glucose regulation, immune system compromise, inflammation, unstable blood pressure, poor sleep cycles, and fatigue. If the low-functioning adrenals continue to be mismanaged, chronic pain, chronic fatigue, allergies, asthma, addiction, and immune or autoimmune system disorders can also set in.

Ovarian Hormones

Ovarian hormones—estrogen, progesterone, and testosterone—all have an important role in regulating your physical, mental, and psychological health, too. Your ovarian hormones interact and regulate mood, metabolism, cognition, sexual function, fertility, weight regulation, sleep cycles, and emotional well-being. And the important thing to remember here is that all these hormones are dynamically affected by high levels of stress. When your hormones are out of balance from high stress, you can feel moody and unable to concentrate, or suffer from premenstrual syndrome (PMS), insomnia, wakefulness, hair loss, headaches, rage, irritability, sore breasts, irregular cycles, uterine fibroids, ovarian cysts, and more.

Thyroid Hormones

Thyroid hormones are also sensitive to high recurrent stress levels. The production of the active thyroid hormone T3 is dependent on its conversion from another compound in your body called T4. But if your cortisol levels are not optimal, this conversion process can be hindered, leading to low thyroid symptoms, or hypothyroidism. Weight gain, dry skin, puffy eyes, brittle nails, hair loss, low mood, afternoon exhaustion, insomnia, brain fog, irregular menstrual bleeding, inflammation, enlarged thyroid, and elevated cholesterol are all symptoms of a low-functioning thyroid.

Brain Transmitters

Your neurotransmitters play a vital role in overseeing nearly every system in your body. They can affect such things as weight regulation, sleep patterns, appetite, perception of pain, sense of well-being, mood, and mental performance. When your neurotransmitters are out of balance, numerous physical and psychological problems can occur. Those with a neurochemical imbalance from stress, for example, have a much higher rate of drug, alcohol, nicotine, caffeine, sugar, and carbohydrate addiction than the rest of the population.

Nervous System

Even the physical structures in your nervous system can be negatively affected and altered with prolonged, unmanaged stress. Many women today tend to operate from a place of activation or, fight or flight (a mode of the sympathetic system) rather than the ideal place of relax, repair, and regenerate (the parasympathetic system).

As a general rule, we need more time in the parasympathetic mode for our bodies to be able to repair themselves. Spending most of our waking hours going full speed down the sympathetic nervous system path without any time for repair and rejuvenation leads to physical and mental side effects due to being in constant activation. This is exhausting to your brain and ultimately leads to a weakened overall nervous system.

THE COST OF STRESS

Most women are dealing with way too many demands in their lives. They are working too many hours and managing too many tasks at work and at home. Women are juggling chores, racing from one thing to the next, and exposing themselves to overstimulation—especially with their phones by constantly moving between emails, texts, and talking. Women's bodies are not wired for this type of excessive hyperstimulation, and in time, without the right tools, they will show signs of breaking down.

These days, medical offices are flooded with women feeling the physical ailments of stress—high blood pressure, fatigue, insomnia, anxiety, breast and uterine problems, and allergies. And the fundamental problem with these visits is that the medical community is not paying attention to what is needed to treat the entire female system with regard to stress-induced problems. This is primarily because medical physicians and practitioners are trained to treat the acute problem and not the underlying condition as it pertains to stress. There is a breakdown in the system by which stress is not recognized as the culprit or treated as such.

What's bothersome about this pervasive view in the medical community is that studies have shown stress is responsible in some way for a whopping 70 to 90 percent of all medical office visits.[3] And women are 75 percent more likely than men to suffer from stress-related depression or anxiety issues.[4] Fortunately, doctors are starting to take notice because of the alarming spike in the incidence of reported stress, the climbing rates of stress-related health problems, and nearly half of all women seeking medication to treat stress-related symptoms. These statistics are hard to ignore. Many women report that they find themselves obsessing over work or responsibilities to the point where they make themselves sick and anxious. Irritable bowels, racing heart, headaches, jaw clinching, back pain, anxiety, depression, high blood pressure, exhaustion, and sleeplessness are all caused by high levels of stress.

In a perfect world, doctors would analyze their patients by stepping back and looking at the entire person, rather than just targeting one particular problem (such as lack of sleep) and prescribing something for it. If a patient were not sleeping and the whole-system approach were used, it might be evident with testing and symptom evaluation that she had

---

3   "America's #1 Health Problem," American Institute of Stress, https://www.stress.org/americas-1-health-problem/.

4   Paul R. Albert, "Why Is Depression More Prevalent in Women?" *Journal of Psychiatry and Neuroscience* 40, no. 4 (2015): 219–221, doi: 10.1503/jpn.150205.

unmanaged stress. This unmanaged stress causes an overactive brain at night, increasing her cortisol and keeping her from sleeping.

The treatment for unmanaged stress is obviously different from simply prescribing a sleeping pill for an inability to sleep and would more likely lead to a long-term fix. Treating the body as a whole and addressing any area that is draining the system will ultimately help you recover more effectively and quickly. You need more than a Band-Aid, which is pretty much what a sleeping pill would be in this instance.

Women seeking medical attention for their stress-related symptoms (though they usually do not know they are stress related) will more often than not leave their doctors' offices with a prescription to treat their specific symptoms rather than having testing done to identify and treat the underlying condition. The number of antidepressant, antianxiety, blood pressure, pain relief, attention deficit, and gut medications written daily in medical offices are continuing to rise primarily for this reason.

And the problem with using medication to treat stress-induced conditions is that these medications often produce harmful side effects that may further compromise your ability to manage stress. These new ailments must also eventually be treated with more medications, each with their own side effects. (Are you sensing a cycle here?) This is why more women are now prescribed multiple medications than ever before.[5]

An example of this pattern of bad prescribing is the use of antidepressants: These medications lower testosterone levels in women, creating more anxiety, weight gain, irritability, low sex drive, and—amazingly—*depression!* (Now *that's* depressing!)

This isn't all your doctor's fault, though. Most medical practitioners, who are already pushed for time in the office, are finding it impossible to figure out what to do with many patients who have multifaceted stress

---

5   Laura A. Pratt, Debra J. Brody, and Qiuping Gu, "Antidepressant Use in Persons Aged 12 and Over: United States, 2005–2008," Centers for Disease Control and Prevention, NCHS Data Brief, no. 76, October 2011, https://www.cdc.gov/nchs/products/databriefs/db76.htm.

symptoms. Many doctors and practitioners have never heard of adrenal hypofunction. Nor do they know how stress interconnects with the endocrine system, the brain, and the nervous system or what to do about it. Ironically, we continue to churn out mounds of research on how high levels of stress affect nearly every area of our body,[6] but these never seem to reach our medical providers. Maybe it's time to connect the dots. Fortunately, hormone specialists and functional medicine physicians and practitioners are continuing to educate their patients on the underlying problems associated with stress and how to treat them.

Stress that remains untreated in women with families not only takes its toll on them but on their families as well, and the cost is significant. The most pressing problem of dual-income families is not money, but the problem of managing extremely hectic family schedules and adjusting spousal duties. Many women are currently juggling full-time careers, household chores, child-rearing, and care of aging parents. Moreover, women naturally pick up the slack and are usually the first to jump into the middle of a problem to solve it. They are often the ones picking up sick kids from school and juggling appointments.

We do all of this because we can. Because we are amazing. But no woman is invincible, and we need to start recognizing our own needs and limitations. I believe it is time that we become advocates for our own health. Brilliant women need to learn how stress is woven into nearly every area of our bodies and minds, to understand the triggers for stress, and to adopt a vigilant self-care plan that will eliminate the need for medications and help us age well while continuing to work and raise children with a revitalized spirit and rejuvenated body.

I know you are ready to learn what it takes to reverse burnout. Clearly, you're not ready to throw in the towel because you are reading this book.

6   Sheldon Cohen, Denise Janicki-Deverts, William J. Doyle, Gregory E. Miller, Ellen Frank, Bruce S. Rabin, and Ronald B. Turner, "Chronic Stress, Glucocorticoid Receptor Resistance, Inflammation, and Disease Risk," *PNAS* 109, no. 16, 5995–5999, doi: 10.1073/pnas.1118355109.

And because it is part of your DNA to be better (or the best). This book will teach you how to get back to the "old you"—only this time, you will be wiser, more strategic, and better equipped with calculated boundaries on how you live your life and manage yourself.

At the end of the day, life is stressful; there is no doubt about it. It would be impossible to eradicate stress completely, and that wouldn't even be a good idea. A certain level of stress is healthy and necessary. Instead, the solution to overcoming burnout lies in reducing as much unnecessary stress as possible and adopting a highly effective, self-care plan to cope with the stress that cannot be removed. Beating burnout requires you to be introspective and step into your most authentic self, and that involves confronting beliefs and mind-sets that are not working for you anymore in order to come up with a new plan that will allow you to reach the highest level of success in all areas of your life, all while feeling content and energized. Fortunately for you, this book will teach you exactly that.

FAST TRACK: COMBATING BURNOUT

Let's face it: We are too busy for a 17-page self-help plan to get back on track. The following is a list of steps to make changes *today* to immediately stop the negative physical and mental side effects of stress. I want you to be successful, and this is the best place to start.

- Take the burnout quiz.

- Check the symptom list that follows to identify the current symptoms you may be experiencing.

- Identify the area of your life where you are struggling the most (like sleep) and immediately read that chapter in this book today.

- Apply one or two fast-track steps from that chapter you have read to your upcoming week.

- Make a plan today to engage in one of the following activities this week: meditation, massage, laughing with a friend, relaxing or walking in nature, sleeping in or taking a nap, nurturing your soul by establishing a way to connect and be quiet, or journaling. Each one of these activities will move you out of activation of the sympathetic nervous system (plugged in) to the parasympathetic (recovery) system, creating a feeling of being "unplugged" and calm. Taking this first step will produce amazing results if you commit to doing it regularly, be it weekly or daily.

- Make a plan on your calendar to map out the chapters of this book, reading at least one chapter per week. Then, create a follow-up plan to implement at least one fast-track step into your daily routine.

- Begin each week by writing one thing in your calendar, phone, or journal that you love about yourself or that makes you feel good about yourself. Don't overthink it.

- This week, start repeating the mantra, "Now is the time for me. I am putting a plan together for better balance and success in all areas of my life."

Your journey begins now. I'm so excited for you. The list that follows showcases the classic burnout symptoms in women. Go through the list and put a checkmark by those symptoms you are experiencing or have experienced recently. This process will help connect you to your body and allow you to hone in on the treatment plans in this book that will address your most pressing symptoms.

CLASSIC BURNOUT SYMPTOMS

....

- ○ Chronic fatigue

- ○ Insomnia

- ○ Forgetfulness/impaired concentration

- ○ Chest pain, heart racing, palpitations

- ○ Shortness of breath—feelings of anxiety

- ○ Dizziness, fainting

- ○ Headaches

- ○ Compromised immune system (frequently ill)

- ○ Loss of appetite or sugar/starch cravings

- ○ Anxiety/tension/constant worry

- ○ Depression/unexplained sadness

- ○ Anger/irritability/rage

- ○ Loss of enjoyment

- ○ Pessimism

- ○ Isolation/detachment

- ○ Hopelessness/apathy

- ○ Lack of productivity

....

Now that you have taken the initial steps to combating burnout, I want to leave you with a little inspiration so you can see how other brilliant women, like you, have gone from wipeout to recovery. In this story you will meet Jamie C., a type-A, executive rock star and a one-of-a-kind woman. Her story might sound familiar to you.

Classic Burnout Success Story

Jamie came to my office six years ago. She was a marketing executive who worked more than 50 hours a week. She was 42 years old and had two children and a husband who worked full time as a sales manager. She was an overachiever in every sense of the word. She sat in my office desperate for answers as we went over her hormone profile and symptom list. She had always been able to manage multiple projects and tasks seamlessly with her perfectly executed to-do lists, maintaining her roles as a mother, wife, daughter, sister, friend, house manager, coach, and business executive. Others, including her family, thought she could pull off anything.

But it was evident that Jamie had hit the proverbial wall. She was consumed with brain fog, irritability, fatigue, cravings, weight gain, exhaustion, anxiety attacks, PMS, irregular periods, and repeated wakefulness at night. She was suffering from classic burnout. But she could not afford to feel this way. She had worked hard to get to the level she was at and did not want to suddenly show weakness or an inability to perform.

Jamie came to me for help, and as we reviewed her labs and made a plan for her recovery, she decided there were things she must change to continue juggling so many different roles.

Her game plan included

- Correcting her female imbalance with natural hormones

- Correcting her low thyroid levels with medication

- Correcting her anxiety with nutritional supplements

- Supporting brain chemistry with amino acids, targeting her low levels for optimal mood support

- Correcting her morning ritual by starting her day with 30 minutes of exercise, 10 minutes of meditation, a higher nutrient shake for her breakfast on the go, planning lunch and dinner, and leaving the home prepared with food and supplements

- Letting go of two activities that she didn't need to continue doing

- Implementing an action plan for "asking for help"

- Letting go of three things that were robbing her of happiness and replacing them with three things that she loved to do that kept her creative side optimized

In 90 days Jamie was 70 percent better. She had renewed energy; no PMS; regular menstrual cycles; no more anxiety; no afternoon drops in her energy; a full, uninterrupted seven hours of sleep at night; less irritability with the kids and husband; and a sense that she could handle her workload much easier.

But we both new she could be even better. So, at the 90-day mark, we reviewed her new lab tests for ovarian, thyroid, and adrenal hormones, tested brain chemicals, and proceeded to adjust her hormones again, while implementing a fat-reduction plan to help her lose the 20 pounds she had gained by drinking mochas and wine (which she had used to self-medicate).

We also optimized her supplement plan and incorporated a new routine for overall life balance, working mostly on clearing the negative mind-set that was still zapping her reserves. And now, I'm happy to report that Jamie has not only recovered 100 percent, but she has also been continuing her brilliance in all areas of her life for six years. She is successful in all areas of her life and feels supported and energetic. And you can, too.

2

Adrenals in Action . . . or *Not*!: Stress Gland Meltdown—the Beginning of the End!

"We need to change the delusion that we need to burn out in order to succeed."

—ARIANNA HUFFINGTON

In this chapter we're going to discuss adrenal fatigue, how it affects the body, and what you can do to prevent it. The quiz below will help to answer that, and may likely bring to light your current state of burnout, also known as *adrenal fatigue*.

QUIZ: DO YOU HAVE ADRENAL FATIGUE?

1. Do you have trouble waking up in the morning? Y/N
2. Do you need caffeine to get going in the morning or throughout the day? Y/N
3. Are you gaining weight around your belly? Y/N

4. Do you get colds/flu easily or sick often? Y/N

5. Do you have low thyroid symptoms despite normal tests? Y/N

6. Are you sensitive to sugars, starches, or alcohol and have a more severe reaction to these substances but still crave them? Y/N

7. Have you developed anxiety, nervousness, or a feeling of panic that you have not always had? Y/N

8. Have you been diagnosed with uterine fibroids, ovarian cysts, polycystic ovarian syndrome (PCOS), or fibrocystic breasts? Y/N

9. Do you feel wired but tired and unable to relax? Y/N

10. Do you wake up in the middle of the night with your mind or heart racing? Y/N

11. Has it become more difficult to manage deadlines and juggle multiple projects? Y/N

12. Do you get lightheaded when you stand up? Y/N

13. Do you fly off the handle at little things more than you used to? Y/N

14. Do you lack interest in sex? Y/N

15. Do you need to eat to prevent low blood sugar episodes (frequent snacking)? Y/N

16. Do you hit the wall in the afternoon? Are you dead tired by 7 p.m. but sometimes get a second wind later in the evening? Y/N

17. Are your PMS, menopause, or perimenopause symptoms getting worse? Y/N

18. Do you have heavy bleeding or irregular cycles more than you used to? Y/N

19. Do you have unexplained hair loss? Y/N

20. Do you crave salty foods? Y/N

21. Does your heart race during the day? Y/N

22. Are you scattered and losing your focus? Y/N

23. Do you have pain in your back or neck or the middle of your butt for no reason? Y/N

24. Do you feel better for a short period of time after eating? Y/N

25. Are you easily startled? Y/N

26. Do you get rattled under pressure, perhaps more than you used to? Y/N

27. Are you developing more sensitivities to medications, supplements, or foods or developing allergies, skin problems, rashes, hives, or itchy skin? Y/N

28. Is your body temperature off? Do you have cold hands and feet or a warm, flushed face? Y/N

If you answered yes to more than 10 of these questions above, it is likely you have adrenal dysfunction and a compromised stress syndrome, often referred to as hypothalamic-pituitary-adrenal (HPA) axis syndrome, or adrenal fatigue.

Hypothalamic-pituitary-adrenal (HPA) axis probably sounds scary, but trust me, there are plenty of simple ways to get your body on the right track. Before we begin dealing with problems with the adrenal glands, though, we need to go through a simple overview of what these glands do and why they are so important.

THE AMAZING ADRENAL STRESS MANAGEMENT SYSTEM

The adrenal glands are your body's hormonal backbone and the linchpin in the feedback loop coordinating nearly every hormone in your body. These yellow glands are powerful little suckers, located on top of your kidneys, weighing in at ¼ ounce and measuring only 1 ½ inches long. Amazingly, despite their diminutive size, they manufacture more than 50 lifesaving hormones and steroids that interface with nearly every bodily function we have—many of which are essential to life itself. Each adrenal gland has two parts, the outer cortex and the inner medulla, both of which produce hormones that are integral to the body's stress management system, including epinephrine, cortisol, DHEA (dehydroepiandrosterone), progesterone, and testosterone.

The Adrenal Cortex and Medulla

The adrenal cortex produces three types of hormones: mineralocorticoids, glucocorticoids, and androgens. Mineralocorticoids (such as aldosterone) help regulate blood pressure, hydration, salt-water ratios, and electrolyte balance. Glucocorticoids (like cortisol) regulate metabolism, blood sugar, digestion, and the immune system. And, last but not least, androgens are the molecules that convert to fully functioning sex hormones, like testosterone.

The medulla, on the other hand, manufactures adrenaline, which gives your body the ability to quickly respond in stressful situations. It gives you that feeling as if you drank a pot of coffee in a single gulp, only naturally. To achieve that effect, adrenaline stimulates your heart, ensures that all parts of your body are getting blood, and converts glycogen into glucose in your liver to prepare your body to manage any stress that might come your way. Clearly these hormones are integral to managing stress, and, since our adrenals produce many of the hormones that are responsible for keeping us alive and balanced as well, it is in our best interest to understand how we can preserve and support these little powerhouses (or in some cases bring them back to life).

Fight-or-Flight Response

Your adrenal glands are part of a system that starts in the hypothalamus (in the upper brain), which connects to the pituitary gland (in the midbrain), which in turn sends signals to the adrenals to produce hormones that get your body mobilized to manage incoming stress. This system is called the HPA axis, after the glands involved in the signal, and is the heart of the body's stress response. This chemical reaction we all have built into our incredibly complex, highly integrative systems is quite interesting when you understand how it works.

Most people have heard of the fight-or-flight response. It's that jolt of energy you feel at the crest of a roller coaster or when the caller ID on your phone reads *Mom*. But to put it clinically, fight or flight is the way your brain perceives, your nervous system activates, and your adrenal stress system prepares your body to react to incoming danger or threats. This multisystem response to danger is also the same system that manages day-to-day encounters with high stress.

The flight-or-fight process starts with a perceived or real stress. Then, your brain registers the incoming threat, which could be something as common as waking up late for work, an argument with your spouse that left you angry and undone, being wrongly accused of something, or constant financial strain.

Once the high-stress signal is sent, your HPA axis system is activated. This survival mechanism extends into the entire hormonal system via the HPA axis, which ultimately protects you from harm by sounding alarms that alert you to get away and move faster. These signals in your body raise glucose levels, elevate your heart rate, and speed up impulses. (Have you ever heard yourself talking when you are stressed? Perhaps you speak more quickly or louder than normal?) When this system is activated, your body is put into survival mode and is suddenly capable of some pretty amazing things. The HPA axis is incredibly effective at mobilizing all your internal resources to help you physically manage stress by:

- Pumping glucose into your bloodstream to create extra sugar in case you need it for quick movements (think running from a tiger)

- Breaking down fat and muscle to mobilize needed glucose for the perceived (or actual) emergency

- Downloading insulin into your bloodstream to help regulate the extra glucose that is now on board (which can lead to fat storage)

- Constricting blood vessels (increased blood pressure and heart rate)

- Directing energy away from daily body functions and metabolism and slowing digestion down (gut problems and weight gain)

- Slowing down cell regeneration (accelerated skin aging)

- Interrupting fertility (missed ovulation, infertility, lack of progesterone—the mood/calm hormone)

- Downregulating your immune system (frequent illnesses)

- Constricting vessels in the brain's blood support (scattered thinking and lack of focus)

These system changes occur as a part of the fight-or-flight response so your body can adequately focus on managing the actual or perceived stressful incident. When the perceived stress dissipates (in a normal situation), the extra blood sugar gets swept up into your cells by insulin. Then, your blood vessels relax, blood flow returns to your gut and reproductive organs, your heart rate slows down, and your body recovers. Soon, the HPA axis returns to its normal state but not if you have reached burnout.

PLUGGED IN 24/7

The body's sophisticated response to stress is nothing short of a miracle. But the reality is that we "overachiever superwomen stress junkies" spend quite a bit of time being plugged in and in fight-or-flight mode, maneuvering strategically between one tense situation to the next. In these instances, our bodies become a ticking time bomb. While our bodies are meant to react to perceived stress occasionally, they are clearly not capable of withstanding longer periods of fight or flight without some sort of breakdown. Think about it: You wouldn't expect a car to run at top speed 100 percent of the time without its engine exploding, so why do we expect it of our bodies?

This elaborate stress response, with multiple internal alarms going off, typically occurs regularly throughout the day for most brilliant women. I can give you hundreds of examples of women stressed out from the moment they wake up until they are finally able to throw themselves in bed at night. This constant state of activation and overstimulation requires your body's continuous effort to preserve and restore your adrenal glands. This is incredibly taxing on your adrenals and causes your entire system to become sluggish, which in turn leaves you depleted and imbalanced, with less cortisol and female hormone production, creating a myriad of symptoms that turn your whole world upside down.

When you are in this state, your adrenals slow down on the production of lifesaving hormones and steroids, like cortisol. This eventually leads to exhaustion and an inability to cope. Your body is sending you the strong message to slow down for your own survival. While adrenal dysfunction used to be rare, it is now all too common because of our lack of relaxation, our excessive hurriedness, and the constant overstimulation to our brain and nervous system. Emotional fatigue is coupled with bad habits, such as smoking; excessive intake of sugars or starches, artificial ingredients, and additives; excessive caffeine consumption; and not sleeping enough.

Now that we know what happens to our system when we are faced with high levels of stress, it might be a good idea to focus on what happens when this kind of strain on our bodies goes on for longer periods of time.

WHAT IS ADRENAL FATIGUE?

At its most basic, adrenal fatigue is a phenomenon characterized by a disruption in the adrenal glands' ability to make cortisol in the right amounts at the right times in response to stress. It is a process that evolves with a gradual onset that is triggered when your nervous system, physical body, adrenal glands, and brain cannot keep up with the tremendous amount of ongoing daily stressors. This can occur because of a single stressful incident (diagnosis of cancer, loss of a loved one, divorce, sick child, financial devastation) or because of prolonged stress (excessive hurriedness, overworking, overeating, consuming sugar or alcohol, chronic pain, sleeplessness, under relaxing, and overachieving). These can lead to a breakdown of signals in the body and underproduction of necessary hormones, including cortisol, estradiol, progesterone, testosterone, and thyroid hormones and neurochemicals, such as serotonin, dopamine, GABA (gamma-aminobutyric acid), and endorphins.

Adrenal fatigue affects nearly every bodily function. In many cases, the adrenal glands shrink, producing fewer and fewer of the hormones needed for your daily get-up-and-go. With adrenal fatigue, the HPA axis loop from your brain to your adrenals and back to your brain becomes sluggish and dysfunctional. A message to begin your body's fight-or-flight response is sent from your brain, but your compromised adrenals do not produce enough cortisol to alert your brain to stop releasing more signaling hormones, thus compromising your entire system. What's worse is that your endocrine system works on feedback loops, and when one system goes down, it calls on another to help out. This is why we often see low thyroid or imbalanced female hormones when adrenal fatigue is present. In other words, this is only the first event in a chain reaction.

Stages of Adrenal Fatigue

There are four primary stages of adrenal fatigue, and each one is associated with a different type of cortisol imbalance. People usually fluctuate between or progress from stage 1 to stage 3 over time. Most women will hover between stages 2 and 3 for many years.

You're probably worried by this point. Your weary adrenals might even be pumping as we speak. But don't panic and skip to the end of the chapter yet, because understanding the differences between these stages and how adrenal fatigue develops is important to knowing where you are in the process and how to treat it. This ultimately should help you determine how seriously you need to take your current life stressors as well as the best strategies to manage them.

The first two stages of adrenal fatigue are the most common, and women recover from these stages easily with intervention and direction. During these phases, neurotransmitters and hormone production can change rapidly, often creating a quick fluctuation between good days and bad days. Each one of the stages presents its own unique symptoms and problems.

THE FOUR STAGES ARE

1. Wired and tired

2. Stressed and depressed

3. Burnout resistance

4. Burnout

STAGE 1: WIRED AND TIRED

This stage describes your body's immediate reaction to a stressful event or series of events. During this first phase, your body can still produce significant amounts of the stress hormones (cortisol) that you need to mount a response and deal with stress physically and mentally without serious consequences. (Oh, to be young again.) Lab testing during this stage would likely show elevated levels of epinephrine (adrenaline), norepinephrine, cortisol, DHEA, and insulin.

During this stage, you will probably feel alert, on top of things, and able to stay up long hours focusing on projects or tasks. Here, you are able to burn the candle at both ends without serious consequences. In this stage, you are high on adrenaline and wired most of the time. With the additional energy, you may find that you have trouble getting to sleep or staying asleep because your brain is racing. This can lead to being tired at night but still wired and not able to rest.

Typically, with the added cortisol and adrenaline, at this stage, you can accomplish more than the average person and it feels good, so you keep doing it. In a way, it's almost addictive—but like most addictive things, it's never good for you in the long run. Many people with intermittent to moderate stress can go in and out of this phase multiple times over the course of their lives and be fine.

STAGE 2: STRESSED AND DEPRESSED

If the intensity of stress continues (life, work, kids, juggling multiple projects, illness, chronic pain, lack of sleep, emotional trauma, etc.), so will your body's reaction to it. With the progression of this high stress, the endocrine triad (adrenals, thyroid, ovaries) and nervous system begin to sound their initial alarms. Although, while your system may be breaking down, at this point, you are still quite able to produce the necessary hormones that you need to combat and manage the physical and mental side effects of stress.

During this phase, your DHEA and testosterone and progesterone levels are likely to fall. This occurs when high stress causes the hormones normally produced to be put on hold to divert the energy to manufacturing lifesaving hormones like cortisol. With the progression of stage 2, the likely side effects are daytime fatigue, dependence on stimulants in the morning and throughout the day, and feeling the pronounced effect of being physically tired but also unable to relax.

Typically, cortisol will peak early, giving you enough energy to get going in the morning, but its production flattens out and drops later, leaving you tired during the afternoon or early evening. You feel worn out. In this phase, cortisol often spikes at night when you finally sit down to rest. It's as if the adrenal glands are saying, "Awesome, this girl finally slowed down. Now we can make some cortisol." Unfortunately, you do not need cortisol at night; you need it during the day. So, sleep is not restorative, and the cycle of symptoms continue or worsen.

STAGE 3: BURNOUT RESISTANCE

During the burnout resistance phase, your adrenals, nervous system, and brain are forced to continue to focus and manage the present or ongoing high stress. Testosterone, DHEA, progesterone, and often estrogen all become unstable, and their production is interrupted, leaving you with hormonal side effects you may never have experienced before (e.g., PMS, early menopause, ovarian cysts, cystic breasts, headaches). The same precursors that stimulate the production of ovarian hormones also do the same for the adrenal system, so energy is diverted away from making hormones like testosterone and DHEA and moved to the production of cortisol. This mostly has to do with pregnenolone, which is a precursor to both testosterone and cortisol.

During this stage, you can still function, with bouts of energy that are more connected to your resting periods. But your sex drive, energy, and stamina are significantly lower than normal in the morning and throughout the day. You lose muscle mass, gain fat around the belly, lack focus and enthusiasm, and are beginning to feel run down. You may also start developing sensitivities to foods. Female hormone changes are much more dramatic and can cause tender breasts, PMS, early menopausal symptoms, cystic ovaries and breasts, and mood swings. Allergies and skin problems often come into play in this stage, and symptoms like irritable bowel and constipation are often intermittent. You may find yourself reacting to stress negatively, with erratic moods, irritability (with a side of rage), or flying off the handle for no reason.

The worst thing about this stage, though, is that it could go on for months or even years. During this stage, many women go to their doctors, only to be put on birth control, antidepressants, antianxiety medication, and sleeping pills, without any female hormone, thyroid, or adrenal testing to see what is causing all these symptoms. And without the proper treatment, it is all too easy for these women to fall into the deepest and final stage of adrenal fatigue.

STAGE 4: BURNOUT

Burnout simply means that you have been running on empty for too long and your body has had enough. Suddenly, you feel exhausted, regardless of how much sleep you've had. The body has finally run out of ways to manage the burden of prolonged stress, and it can't figure out how to manufacture enough stress hormones when all of the supporting hormones from the ovaries and thyroid are compromised and imbalanced. During this phase, your reserves are depleted. Your cortisol levels drop significantly, leaving you feeling exhausted and without the tools to manage stress physically, mentally, and emotionally. Even with rest, you are unable to stay on top of things as you once were. Lowered cortisol eventually compromises your thyroid function by interfering with the conversion of T4 (storage thyroid) to T3 (active thyroid), leaving you with a slowed metabolism; dry, patchy, itching skin; weight gain; constipation; insomnia; and feeling as if you have hit the proverbial wall. Yeah. Burnout is a bitch.

In addition to all these physical symptoms, in this stage your neurotransmitters are low, leaving you feeling depressed, anxious, occasionally frantic, and craving salt and sugar. Having lost your passion, you couldn't care less about having sex and are irritable and generally disinterested in most everything. This stage can negatively affect every area of your body (see Figure 1.1 in chapter 1).

Since its effects are so widespread, the recovery from this stage likewise takes a multisystem approach. This method entails testing your entire system and coming up with a plan to plug all the "holes" so your body stops draining the necessary hormones you need to recover, and you can get back to who you once were. Yes, that is possible, but it must be handled and approached the correct way and not masked by drugs and the continued frantic lifestyle that got you there in the first place. So put down the chardonnay; it's time to get to work.

Testing for Adrenal Fatigue

The first step is always to get an accurate assessment of the problem, and this means testing. There are several types of testing options to assess and diagnosis adrenal fatigue. I prefer to use a whole-body approach:

- A comprehensive symptom and medical history questionnaire

- Serum (blood) testing for the adrenals, thyroid, and ovarian hormones

- Neurochemical testing to assess possible lower levels in the brain that affect mood

- Full evaluation of all lifestyle habits and patterns with diet, sleep, and current or past stressful events

Cortisol, pregnenolone, DHEA, and testosterone are all hormones that can be tested and are vital to optimal adrenal functioning. The correct testing for adrenal fatigue requires not only blood and saliva testing but also a comprehensive look at the individual woman and her symptoms so a personalized treatment plan can be given. The balance and ratios of these assessments (including laboratory findings and a physical exam) are what the trained medical providers are looking for to determine the stage of fatigue and appropriate treatment plan for anyone presenting with adrenal dysfunction. Every woman is unique and requires a specific treatment plan based on her individual needs.

THE FOLLOWING ARE SOME ADRENAL TESTING OPTIONS:

- Cortisol

- Serum testing

- Saliva testing

- ACTH challenge

- DHEA/cortisol ratio

- 17-hydroxyprogesterone (17-OHP)

- DHEA-S

- Pregnenolone test

- Postural low blood pressure

CORTISOL

Optimally, your cortisol level should be high in the early morning so you can have energy and focus to stay alert and focused, and low at night so you can relax and enjoy deep, restorative sleep. Cortisol has a rhythm that, when optimal, looks like Figure 2.1.

OPTIMAL CORTISOL RHYTHM

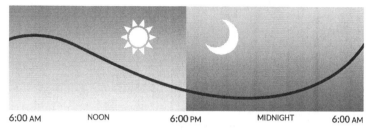

6:00 AM   NOON   6:00 PM   MIDNIGHT   6:00 AM

Cortisol levels are optimal when elevated in the morning to provide focus, concentration, energy and stamina and low at night to promote deep sleep, relaxation and recovery.

REVERSED CORTISOL RHYTHM

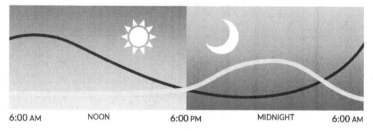

6:00 AM   NOON   6:00 PM   MIDNIGHT   6:00 AM

Cortisol low in the daytime leads to daytime fatigue, weight gain, mood issues, glucose dysregulation, cravings, and the need for stimulants to stay awake. Cortisol rising at night creates a "wired and tired" feeling with trouble getting to sleep and staying asleep. Cortisol production at night leads to low levels the next day

ERRATIC CORTISOL RHYTHM

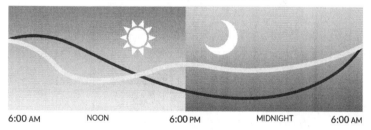

6:00 AM   NOON   6:00 PM   MIDNIGHT   6:00 AM

Cortisol level is normal in the morning, with sharp drops in the afternoon, leading to exhaustion, scattered thinking, low glucose episodes, cravings and mood changes. At night, cortisol rising causes wakefulness and interrupted sleeping patterns.

Figure 2.1: Graph of Varied Cortisol Rhythms

In addition to having a rhythm, cortisol is your "get things done" hormone (unlike adrenaline, which is more of the "panic" hormone). It is secreted to

- Wake you up in the morning

- Turn on your brain for optimal focus

- Get your entire system revved up and ready to tackle the day with energy and focus

- Provide sufficient mobilization of internal resources to help you manage any stress that comes your way

- Power you up during the day to help manage stress more effectively

- Power down at night so you can go into recovery mode and sleep deeply

SERUM TESTING

Serum (blood) testing can be drawn once or multiple times over the course of the same day. It can also be drawn at the exact time of day when a woman feels her worst (like the early morning or possibly in the afternoon). But keep in mind that not all serum tests are created equal. Seeing a medical provider with experience in testing and evaluating stress-related adrenal issues is extremely important because numerous factors should be taken into consideration. Normal ranges on most labs make it confusing for the inexperienced medical provider and patient because these can be misleading. Using optimal ranges and having experience interpreting these tests is vital when diagnosing and treating burnout. Simply being in the normal reference range is not good enough. Furthermore, using the same testing each time is also important so you can more accurately see the progression of your treatment.

SALIVA TESTING

Saliva testing allows you to view the full rhythm of your body's production of cortisol throughout the day by collecting four samples from early morning to late at night. This test allows you to identify the problem time for your hormones. If your cortisol is low in the morning and high at night, this might explain why you're tired during the day and wired at night. If your cortisol is normal in the morning and then drops off sharply at lunch or in the early afternoon, this would explain why you tend to hit a wall later in your day. Saliva testing can be important in diagnosing the exact problem with an abnormal cortisol rhythm.

ACTH CHALLENGE

The adrenocorticotropic hormone (ACTH) challenge test consists of first measuring your baseline cortisol level and then, after having an injection of ACTH, your cortisol is measured again. The injection of ACTH is done to stimulate the production of cortisol (which simulates stress) so a measurement can be taken to reveal how you are compensating for stress physically. If the test shows little elevation, it could suggest a low-functioning adrenal gland, which would require immediate treatment.

DHEA/CORTISOL RATIO

This blood test will show a lower DHEA-to-cortisol ratio in earlier stages of adrenal fatigue. This is because the resources used to make DHEA can be diverted to making more cortisol to manage stress. As adrenal fatigue progresses, both DHEA and cortisol levels begin to fall, but DHEA levels fall faster—thus the lower ratio. This number then helps determine where you might be in the progression of the stages of adrenal hypofunction.

17-HYDROXYPROGESTERONE (17-OHP)

This test is useful, as 17-OHP is a steroid hormone that is a building block for the production of cortisol. With abnormally functioning adrenals, the

17-OHP in your blood is often high due to the fact that your adrenals are struggling to convert it to cortisol, creating elevated blood levels.

DHEA-S

DHEA-S is the most abundant precursor hormone in your body. It is made in the adrenal glands and the brain. When your cortisol levels are high for long periods of time because of stress, resources used to manufacture DHEA are diverted to cortisol, and then DHEA levels drop, causing such side effects as weight gain, accelerated aging, inflammation, and a lowered immune system.

PREGNENOLONE TEST

Pregnenolone, a hormone manufactured by your adrenals, is a precursor to cortisol. Typically, your pregnenolone is low when you have low-functioning adrenals. This can lead to memory and sleep problems. A simple blood test will determine what your levels are.

POSTURAL LOW BLOOD PRESSURE

This test can be done at home or at your doctor's office. During this test, your blood pressure will be taken while lying down, seated, and standing. The normal response in healthy women is that blood pressure should rise immediately upon sitting and then a little more after standing up. If your blood pressure stays the same or even drops after sitting up, or standing up, it could signal a case of low-functioning adrenals.

OPTIMAL ADRENAL RECOVERY

Once you have gone through the appropriate tests and identified your particular dysfunction, it is time to look at treatments. Fortunately, hundreds of supplements are available for treating adrenal dysfunction. The most important factor in choosing from them is simply to know what your needs are through testing and to determine what stage of adrenal fatigue you are in. There are three categories of supplements that you can choose from for adrenal-stress support, starting with the least aggressive and moving up to the more aggressive supplements if a bigger response is needed or your adrenal symptoms are not resolving.

Adaptogens

These are herbs with special properties to help you adapt to stress by normalizing or regulating the adrenal stress response. They will help elevate or lower stress hormones according to your body's need. Adaptogens are excellent choices for stages 1 and 2 of adrenal fatigue. (For a full list of these, see Appendix A.)

Adrenal Glandular Extracts

These are bovine extracts of specific hormones that provide bioavailable building blocks to strengthen your adrenals, hypothalamus, pituitary, and ovaries. These are typically used when rebuilding lower cortisol levels and are a good choice for stages 3 and 4 of adrenal fatigue.

Hydrocortisone

This is a last-resort replacement for cortisol, to help supplement and repair your adrenals' inability to manufacture sufficient levels of cortisol, which can leave you feeling exhausted, in pain, and unable to cope. This is typically appropriate only for stage 4, when all other options have failed. It is available by prescription only.

FAST TRACK: TREATING ADRENAL HYPOFUNCTION

Here it is—what you have so patiently been waiting for. Assuming you fall into one of the categories of adrenal fatigue, or are headed in that direction, I have included a fast-track plan for you to begin reversing the negative effects of a poor cortisol rhythm. Let's get started and give your poor glands a break.

Step 1: Change Your Diet and Timing

Reduce blood glucose spikes and dips by eating the following foods at the suggested times:

BREAKFAST: BETWEEN 7 AND 9 A.M.

Eat high protein and high fat, which will eliminate morning grogginess. This type of breakfast will also stave off afternoon cravings by avoiding heavy carbs in the morning, which tank your energy and fog up your brain. That means no bagels or muffins for breakfast (or donuts—how are those even a breakfast food?). Protein is brain food and will improve your focus and memory for the entire day.

Suggestion: Eggs, mixed greens, and goat cheese, with sesame seeds sprinkled on top.

LUNCH: BETWEEN 11 A.M. AND NOON

Have protein, fat, and light carbs for lunch.

Suggestion: Sliced turkey, feta, apple slices, ten to twelve nuts and seeds on top of greens for a delicious salad. This action-packed meal will keep your glucose from taking a dive. The timing is key here: Do not wait too long to eat. Those with adrenal fatigue need to eat every three to four hours to avoid glucose dumps followed by exhaustion and cravings. Unlike most diets, if you do this one right, you will rarely be hungry.

AFTERNOON SNACK: BETWEEN 3 AND 4 P.M.

Have a snack that includes protein, fat, and light carbs.

Suggestion: Protein bar, Greek yogurt, or protein smoothie with six to eight toasted walnuts or pecans (which are known to help balance cortisol). Add a square of dark chocolate to boost your mood and keep cortisol balanced. But don't get carried away with the chocolate and carbs. So, a huge bowl of pasta and slice of chocolate cake are both out. Sorry.

DINNER: BETWEEN 5 AND 7 P.M.

Include protein and dense carbs in your evening meal.

Suggestion: Quinoa with shrimp or a stir fry; or chicken, veggies, and two to three small, red potatoes. If you have a dinner that has starchy carbohydrates (the opposite of what you have been told), you will boost brain chemicals for mood and sleep.

The goal for optimal treatment with this diet is to remove everything that is making you sick and tired and to instead fill up on foods that help repair your adrenal gland functions. Here are more foods that you should consider eating or snacking on, as they help overcome adrenal insufficiency by being nutrient dense, high in fiber, and low in sugar. Eating them will give you more consistent energy and stamina while supporting hormone balance and adrenal function:

- Coconut

- Olives

- Avocados

- Cruciferous vegetables (cauliflower, broccoli, brussels sprouts)

- Fatty fish (wild-caught salmon)

- Chicken and turkey

- Walnuts and almonds

- Pumpkin, chia, and flax seeds

- Kelp and seaweed

- Celtic or Himalayan sea salt

Step 2: Take Vitamin C

This might be a surprise if you thought vitamin C was just for treating colds and making you feel better about drinking those super-sugary fruit sodas, but, in fact, the highest concentration of vitamin C in the body is stored in the adrenal glands. Vitamin C is utilized by the adrenal glands in the production of cortisol and other adrenal hormones. When you are under stress, your vitamin C levels are rapidly depleted with the production of cortisol and other stress hormones, leading to further weakening of the immune system. The key here is to give your glands what they need by not only eating more foods rich in vitamin C but also by taking higher doses of vitamin C at key times during the day. Foods rich in vitamin C include peppers, strawberries, guavas, kale, spinach, broccoli, oranges, apples, and papaya. Yum!

I recommend ½–1 tsp of vitamin C powder (see Appendix A) mixed in a bottle of water in the morning after breakfast, and ½–1 tsp of vitamin C powder mixed in a bottle of water for lunch time. (You can prefill your bottles in the morning.) This will give you approximately 2,000–4,000 milligrams of vitamin C twice daily at the times you need it the most. This is a higher dose than you would normally take, but, due to your body's increased need for repair, you will use it. You will notice an immediate improvement. And vitamin C powder is less likely to upset your stomach than taking eight to ten capsules per day to get the same dose.

Step 3: Exercise

I'm sure you guessed this was coming, and, trust me, you just gotta do it. But, luckily, in your case, low-impact exercise is going to be better. Walking, yoga, Pilates, and light strength training will serve you better than pounding it out in a spin class or running. Any type of vigorous exercise will leave your adrenals even more taxed because one of the causes of adrenal fatigue is overexercising. If you constantly force yourself to do high-intensity exercise when you are in adrenal fatigue, you will be easily injured or your fatigue will worsen.

Step 4: Take the Right Supplements

Using supplements is one of the best options for recovery. Adding in additional vitamins and herbal adaptogens to support adrenals' optimal functioning will improve your energy, stamina, and quality of sleep. If you are actively in stages 1–4, you might consider this supplement game plan for protecting yourself or reversing the symptoms. (See Appendix A for supplement options.)

ON RISING:
Take two morning-stress-support supplements.

AFTER BREAKFAST:
Take ½–1 tsp of vitamin C power in water and one dropperful of B complex, sublingually.

AT LUNCH:
Take ½–1 tsp of vitamin C powder in water.

BETWEEN LUNCH AND EARLY AFTERNOON:
Take two morning-stress-support supplements.

AT BEDTIME OR ONE HOUR BEFORE:

Take two evening-stress-support supplements. If you wake up during the night, take two more evening-stress-support supplements.

You may also take the following supplements, especially if testing shows low levels:

- High-potency vitamin D (consider a blood test to determine where you are)

- DHEA for energy, stamina, sex drive, and weight control

- Selenium to support the thyroid and for overall energy

- Magnesium to help with sleep, muscle pain, and constipation

- Zinc to improve hormone balance and metabolization of hormones

- Adrenal glandular extracts for stage 3 adrenal fatigue

Step 5: Hydrate

Dehydration is one of the most common problems with adrenal fatigue. Adding a multi–trace mineral supplement will help your body get the water you drink into your cells, which will perk up your mind and system quickly. Adding fresh lemon and Himalayan or Celtic sea salt will also add needed minerals. Overall, drinking water throughout the day will serve you well in the area of energy and brain function.

Step 6: Enjoy Ten Minutes of Silence, Twice Daily

Take ten minutes twice daily to reboot. I still find it weird that I have to tell people to do this, but trust me, this is a serious necessity. Your reboot can be taking a walk outside for ten minutes or sitting in your car with the seat laid back and your eyes closed or even lying down in the back-seat (even better). Please create a plan to take this necessary time, and then make yourself follow through.

When you come home from work, consider taking ten minutes to lie down, or even stop around the block from your house before you enter, to collect yourself and breathe. This will give you so much more recovery and perspective in your daily life. Unplug your brain and engage in belly breathing (where you focus your breath on your belly as you inhale and exhale). This will calm your entire nervous system and create a way for you to repair. This does not include taking a walk while talking and texting or reading a book while sitting in a break room chatting with others. Silence is golden. Breathe from your belly and relax. It will move your nervous system into rest and repair mode. (Brilliant, right?)

Step 7: Get Deep, Restorative Sleep

Diet and sleep are the hallmarks of adrenal fatigue recovery. Research consistently shows that when stressed, our bodies need more sleep.[7] We need a minimum of seven to eight hours of restful sleep per night, even without high stress in our lives. Skimping on sleep handicaps the brain, nervous system, hormonal system, and the body as a whole by robbing it of needed recovery from the previous day and hindering the rejuvenation of hormones and neurochemicals to get you through the next day. If you are not sleeping, I suggest taking high-potency sleep supplements to get your brain turned off and into deep, stage-4 sleep. There are many supplements that help restore sleep and correct bad sleeping habits. You must sleep to keep going, so make this step a top priority.

Getting to sleep before 10 p.m. is a vital part of this. People who go to sleep after 11 p.m. often have surges of cortisol that keep them from going

---

7   "More Sleep Would Make Most Americans Happier, Healthier, and Safer," American Psychological Association, February 2014, https://www.apa.org/research/action/sleep-deprivation.aspx.

to sleep (like a second glass of wine, which is also not recommended). You make vital hormones for recovery, like human growth hormone, between 11 p.m. and 2 a.m., which means being a night owl will set you back and age you like crazy. So, stop working and go to bed.

Some suggestions to get you to sleep earlier include:

- Turn off computers, phones, TVs, or other sensory stimulants thirty to sixty minutes before going to bed. This is the only way to tell your nervous system that you are winding down.

- Take a bath; drop in some lavender oil to optimize your senses for deep relaxation.

- Drink a cup of chamomile tea.

- Do not start doing housework right before bedtime.

- Do not get into an argument with your partner, kids, family, or friends before bedtime.

- Keep your room cool (I recommend 68°F), free of pets, and, if needed, go to the other room if your partner is snoring. Your sleep is too important to miss out on due to loud interruptions.

- Take sleep supplements as needed to get to sleep, and do not let a sleep problem go on without fixing it or getting help to fix it. You will not heal without sleep.

Adrenals in Action Success Story

I have a patient named Jessie, whose story is a true picture of burnout. On top of a demanding work life, she was always on the go with her two teenage girls. Her husband frequently traveled out of town, leaving her with the stress of running a home and parenting as her load to bear. She believed in giving her kids experiences, so every vacation or long weekend was action packed, always leaving her feeling more exhausted when she returned to work. She was sleeping about five hours per night and trying to eat a no-carb diet to lose weight. She was hungry most of the time and had no success in losing weight. She started noticing constant pains in her hips and buttocks that would grow worse when her stress peaked during the day.

Being the overachiever that she was, she would race home after work to cook dinner, knowing it was the healthiest option for her girls. After dinner, she planned healthy breakfasts and lunches. She also picked up after the kids, did the laundry and the dishes, and, of course, took the dogs on an evening walk.

She would throw herself into bed at night with her laptop to fire off fifty more emails and then hope to God she could sleep. In the morning, she would wake up feeling exhausted. She could tell that her ability to think clearly was fading, which was affecting her job. She had little patience with her kids and was moody, swinging between feeling passionate about her life and work and feeling overwhelmed and depressed. She drank coffee all day to stay awake, and every stressful incident she encountered, especially emotionally charged ones, took everything out of her. She was having recurrent bouts of sickness, premenstrual headaches, a rock-bottom sex drive, and constant sugar cravings. She had no way of giving up any of her mandatory duties in life but also felt as if she couldn't go on doing what she was doing.

Just listening to Jessie's story, it was evident she had stage 3 adrenal hypofunction and was on the edge of stage 4. We immediately began testing and ordered a full hormone, adrenal, thyroid, and stress profile and found that her testosterone was rock bottom, affecting her sex drive, energy, ambition, and focus as well as causing muscle loss and inability to manage stress. Her progesterone level was also very low due to not ovulating (a stress symptom), causing heavy periods, PMS, and head-aches. Her serotonin levels were found to be 50 points below the low end of normal, causing depression, anxiety, and poor quality of sleep. Her morning cortisol level was at the astronomically low level of four at 8 a.m. (Typically, we would see the level at this time around 20, which is high to help you power up for your day.) This helped explain why she felt exhausted even after a full night of sleep.

Additionally, she had elevated insulin levels and low glucose, which were creating cravings, headaches, belly fat, and weight gain. Her thyroid was normal but at the low end for active T3 thyroid, causing increased fatigue, weight gain, mental fogginess, and skin problems. Last, her vita-min D level was low at 12 (optimal is 60), causing further fatigue and recurring sickness.

Jessie knew she needed to make some changes in her life and begin a self-care regimen. So, together, we came up with the following plan.

HER GAME PLAN INCLUDED

- Meeting with our nutritional advisor to overhaul her diet, incor-porating more protein, less fat, and eliminating sugar altogether to help her lose weight

- Eating good carbs in the evening to help boost mood and promote sleep

- Correcting her low levels of testosterone and progesterone with hormone pellet therapy

- Supplementing her nutrition plan with adrenal adaptogens, vitamin D, and B complex for one month through weekly shots and IV ther-apy to jump-start her energy and decrease inflammation

- Starting a walking program of 10–20 minutes a day for stress relief and exercise

- Avoiding saying negative things like "I am so stressed" and replacing them with positive statements like "I choose myself and am ready for better health"

- Getting better sleep by going to bed at 9:00 p.m. and ending all her work by at least 8:30 p.m. so she could let her nervous system switch into sleep mode

Jessie was quite motivated for change, mostly because she was at the end of her rope and didn't want to feel so awful anymore. She began the 12-week overhaul program and lost 20 pounds; most of her belly fat was completely gone. She no longer reported any PMS symptoms, and her premenstrual headaches completely resolved. She had a significant improvement in her sex drive, and finally having satisfying sex also gave her the needed oxytocin boost and softened her feminine side, creating the "lovely feeling" that she thought she had lost. Her relationship with her husband improved dramatically, and she noticed feeling calmer and happier.

She no longer woke up feeling hungover in the morning and noticed her energy upon waking was increased, which activated her brain and body in a much better, healthier way. Her focus and memory improved as she began sleeping more hours. Additionally, her sleep was less interrupted, which improved her mood and overall feeling of well-being. She snapped at her kids about 50 percent less and was much less irritated with everyone around her. She knew she was handling stress better.

Jessie's repeat blood work showed optimal ranges for progesterone and testosterone, serotonin, vitamin D, and cortisol. She was so happy and could hardly believe that her body, mind, and emotions had all changed so dramatically in 12 weeks. Her friends and family told her repeatedly that she seemed happier and more calm and, of course, that she looked amazing.

These are the results I want for all of you. And if you take the time to identify your specific burnout causes and stick with your plan to combat them, I know you can get back to your brilliant self in no time.

3

Hormone Hurricane: Halting the Hormone Havoc . . . Making Your Hormones Your B*tch

"Ignorance is not bliss. Ignorance is devastation.
Ignorance is tragedy. Ignorance is illness."
—JIM ROHN

The endocrine system is insanely complex, so hormonal imbalances can look different from one person to the next. However, some common symptoms that out-of-whack hormones can cause in women are directly related to stress. Take the following quiz to see how your hormones are responding to everyday stress.

QUIZ: ARE YOU IN THE MIDST OF A HORMONE HURRICANE?

1. Have you recently experienced weight gain? Y/N
2. Do you have acne? Y/N

3. Have you experienced an increase in body hair? Y/N

4. Do you have facial hair? Y/N

5. Are you experiencing loss of the hair on your head? Y/N

6. Is your skin thinning? Y/N

7. Do you have brittle hair or nails? Y/N

8. Do you have more belly fat now than you used to have? Y/N

9. Are your eyes puffy? Y/N

10. Do you experience migraines or headaches? Y/N

11. Do you suffer from night sweats? Y/N

12. Do you retain water? Y/N

13. Do you experience hot flashes? Y/N

14. Do you have excessive sugar or salt cravings? Y/N

15. Are you experiencing incontinence? Y/N

16. Do you suffer from dryness, vulvar irritation, or lack of lubrication? Y/N

17. Are you often constipated? Y/N

18. Do you suffer from irritable bowel syndrome or gut problems? Y/N

19. Are you often fatigued or exhausted? Y/N

20. Do you suffer from PMS or early menopause symptoms (even if you are still cycling)? Y/N

21. Do you often have body pain, stiffness, or muscle and joint inflammation? Y/N

22. Do you have a low libido and an inability to climax? Y/N

23. Do you experience anxiety, depression, mood swings, and sadness? Y/N

24. Have you lost your zest or excitement for life? Y/N

25. Do you find it hard to concentrate and stay focused? Y/N

26. Do you worry excessively, and are you unable to manage stress? Y/N

27. Have you lost your stamina and drive? Y/N

If you marked yes to at least four of the above symptoms, you likely have some sort of hormone imbalance that is often linked to stress. You may want to get tested and treated by a hormone expert.

....

If you have been reading everything up to this point, it should be abundantly clear to you by now that whatever is going on with your stress glands and with your life in general will directly affect your hormones. And in the lives of brilliant women suffering from burnout, the sex hormones are the keys to just about everything. It's sufficient to say that your female hormones—estrogen, progesterone and testosterone—pretty much run your entire system and directly interact with the thyroid, stress glands, brain chemicals, gut, nervous system, and brain. (Oh, is that all?) Therefore, it's worth figuring out any imbalance that may exist with these hormones that may be causing you daily distress.

Problems with these hormones can often go overlooked because they tend to be things we attribute to normal aging. But if you are feeling fat, frazzled, overwhelmed at times, and exhausted, figuring out if you have a hormone imbalance is as simple as taking a blood test. For more than 27 years now, I have listened to women tell me that they were told by their doctors how what they were feeling was normal and just age related or stress related. Well, I am here to tell you that while stress may be the culprit, stress can kill you, so how you feel now should never be dismissed as just stress.

HORMONAL HIGHS AND LOWS

Hormones are essential to life. They are chemical connectors to the brain, muscles, sex organs, and virtually every part of the body. If you were suddenly left without the intricate communication in your body conducted via hormones, you would die—pretty much immediately. As it is, even a missed message, a broken connection, or an unclear communication from one hormone to another can cause an imbalance, upsetting the whole shebang. As early as a woman's midthirties, a small drop in estrogen or progesterone, or a break in her ovulation cycle can cause a domino effect of mood instability, weight gain, skin problems, and many other changes. Even though nearly every woman knows she will eventually experience menopause, these changes can come as unpleasant surprises. In addition, diet, stress, sleep patterns, environmental toxins, and genetics can create complete hormone chaos that may leave you feeling terrible for years to come.

This is the hard truth about life as a woman. Something happens, whether it's stress, diet, or medications—or a genetic predisposition—that throws your system for a loop, and afterward your hormones either revert to a normal state or they don't. It depends on how healthy you are to begin with. The key is to take care of yourself so you're not as susceptible to these inevitable hormone fluctuations. Even though much of what happens in life is beyond your power, you *can* control what you eat, how much you exercise, how many hours you sleep, and whether you use vitamin and herbal supplements. In menopause (or early menopause), some women adjust to the chronically low levels and others do not.

HORMONES AND THE ADRENAL GLANDS

Stress and the adrenal glands play a huge role in hormone balance. After all, the adrenal glands are responsible for producing estrogen, progesterone, and testosterone during perimenopause and menopause. Chronic or sustained high levels of stress is often the only source of the hormone imbalance women feel. Once your body gets into a stress cycle, it will begin using the progesterone and testosterone in your system and transforming them into cortisol, the stress hormone. When this happens, your stress system is literally stealing from your sex hormone system, throwing off the balance and creating even more symptoms, making you even more stressed. (Oh God, even thinking about it is stressing me out!)

But worsening stress is only the beginning. Sustained levels of stress create hormone imbalances that, in turn, trigger fat storage, weight gain, and many other unwanted symptoms, like PMS, acne, painful breasts, irritable bowels, migraines, exhaustion, loss of sex drive, cellulite, irregular periods, premature wrinkles, and burnout. Yikes! Your hormones dictate virtually every part of your life—from your state of mind to your behavior, body shape, eating habits, sleep, and your reaction to stress. When you are facing ongoing high stress, your adrenals need support to keep the most vital functions going, and they will gladly steal from your female hormones to get it.

Your body is fully aware of the fact that the fight-or-flight hormones are needed to help you manage your daily dose of stress, and its priority is the adrenal glands (not the ovarian hormones). You cannot live without cortisol, but you can survive with a female hormone imbalance. (You'll just feel like crap.) The goal for treating this is to balance your hormones. Your stress glands will then be more supported and will stop stealing resources from your ovaries so you will have little to no symptoms of hormone decline.

THE IMPORTANCE OF BALANCED HORMONES

Hormones are pretty incredible. They serve as messengers between body systems to regulate behavior, digestion, metabolism, respiration, tissue function, sleep, stress, growth, movement, reproduction, and mood. Hormones tell your body when you are hungry, sleepy, stressed, or getting a little frisky. They also tell you when to stop eating, wake up, calm down, move forward, slow down, or even run for cover.

The hormones produced in our ovaries, thyroid, and adrenals are constantly interacting, and we must pay attention to what their needs are in order to feel our best and stay in the game longer while performing at the highest level. Estrogen (estradiol), progesterone, and testosterone are the three main female sex hormones. (We call them sex hormones, as they are produced in the ovaries, the sex gland.) There are many other hormones in the body, but few have the same type of clearly seen impact as these primary sex hormones, especially for women.

Sex hormones control the most influential processes in the body, such as pregnancy, puberty, regulating the menstrual cycle, menopause, hair growth, skin condition, complexion, mood, muscle storage, fat accumulation... I could go on. It may also surprise you to hear that men and women have the same sex hormones, only in different ratios. The tricky part about female hormones, though, is that they function differently in certain areas of the body. They can complement each other and often function as opposites. This is precisely the reason that the correct ratios with hormones should be maintained and amended if they are not in balance.

So now that you have some idea about how complex your endocrine system is, as well as how important maintaining the balance of hormones in your body can be, let's get into the nitty-gritty work of determining whether or not you are dealing with a hormone imbalance before we tackle how to fix it.

THE CLASSIC SYMPTOMS OF A HORMONE HURRICANE
INCLUDE FEELING:

- **Bitchy:** Loss of progesterone due to lack of ovulation, itself due to excessive stress interfering with ovulation

- **Fat:** Imbalance between estrogen and progesterone leading to estrogen dominance, which creates glucose instability and insulin resistance (belly fat)

- **Frazzled:** Plummeting levels of testosterone due to poor functioning, overtaxed adrenals, and the conversion of testosterone to life-saving cortisol leaves women feeling frantic, frazzled, and out of control with no focus.

- **Fatigued:** Lack of progesterone (mood/sleep hormone), dysrhythm of cortisol, and estrogen dominating the cycle lead to shallow sleep, wakefulness, stimulation of the brain at night, and less than optimal thyroid output.

Nobody wants to live in a hormone hurricane—so how are you supposed to get better? The root cause of these issues is nearly always hormonal imbalance, and you must first connect the right hormone with the exact symptoms to even begin getting back to your old self and feeling great. Let's examine each sex hormone and the consequences of its dysfunction to help you hone in on which ones might need balancing. But first, a word about where these imbalances come from.

WHAT CAUSES A HORMONAL IMBALANCE?

The causes of hormone imbalances are pretty unfair because they are often self-induced. Stress has a huge influence on hormonal imbalances.

The stress on your hormones from not sleeping well, eating a high sugar or starch diet, not getting enough minerals and nutrients, or ongoing poor lifestyle habits such as excessive drinking can cause hormonal imbalances. For most people, that's just called living your life, but we brilliant women can always do better. There are also a number of outside influences to watch out for that can lead you down the path of hormone upheaval. These include

Environment

- Chronic stress

- Chemical exposure from foods, lotions, and shampoos

- A sedentary lifestyle with overstimulation from computers, phones, and electronics

- Artificial light

- Exposure to plastics and contaminants

Diet

- Not enough fatty acids (good fats)

- Artificial ingredients, toxins, hormones, and preservatives in the foods we eat

- Not enough fiber

- Lack of vitamin C, B complex, magnesium, or zinc

- Excessive candida in the gut (compromising the absorption of nutrients and vitamins)

- Too much soy

- Excessive alcohol intake

- Too many unhealthy fats

- Processed foods (man-made foods)

- Overeating or undereating

- Poor eating habits as a vegan (e.g., eating too many carbs)

Lifestyle

- Lack of sleep (less than 7 hours of good stage 4 restorative sleep)

- Not breathing fully

- Little or no exercise (no outlet for the "stress steam")

- Overexercising or competing without proper self-care

The Liver and Toxic Chemicals

A big factor in whether or not you will develop a hormone imbalance in your life boils down to how you treat your poor liver. Alcohol, medications, chemicals, heavy metals, and other toxins in our environment (or red Solo cups) burden the liver. This is a problem because the liver is the most important organ for breaking down excess estrogen and getting it out of your system. A liver that's overloaded is sluggish and will create an environment that slows down detoxification, resulting in a hormone imbalance often in the form of an excess accumulation of estrogen.

Speaking of things that are toxic for you: fat. High percentages of body fat mean high percentages of toxins being stored in the fat cells. But even more importantly for women, excess body fat means the body will store more estrogen, which leads to low testosterone and more fat gain and muscle loss. There is also an enzyme known as aromatase in the fat tissue that converts testosterone *into* estrogen, further complicating the imbalance and fat gain.

Making things worse, when estrogen is elevated and out of balance with progesterone and testosterone levels, it interacts with insulin (the fat-storage hormone). Insulin is needed to get glucose from your blood into your cells, but when estrogen is elevated, it can cause fluctuations in your blood sugar level and upset your insulin factory (the pancreas). If the production of insulin is not kept in check, your cells can become less insulin sensitive. As a result, the sugar in your blood cannot enter your cells to be used for fuel, forcing the body to store it as fat (creating yet another vicious cycle).

As we age, our hormones decline naturally. The graph below shows how hormones, particularly progesterone and testosterone, begin to drop off at age 30. And as women age under the influence of prolonged stress, this drop-off is more severe. If you add in poor lifestyle with stress, lack of exercise, excessive body fat, a toxic liver, and a round of nightly alcohol, you will likely have the perfect formula for hormones gone wild. This is why hormone imbalance symptoms in younger women are becoming more common.[8]

---

8   Burcu Ceylan and Nebahat Özerdoğan, "Factors Affecting Age of Onset of Menopause and Determination of Quality of Life in Menopause," *Turkish Journal of Obstetrics and Gynecology* 12, no. 1: 43–49, doi: 10.4274/tjod.79836.

The Decline of Hormones with Age

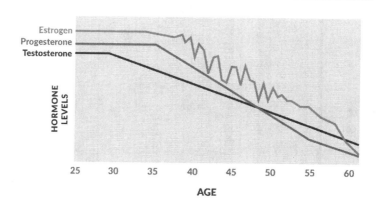

Figure 3.1: Graph of Sex Hormone Decline with Age

SPECIFIC HORMONE IMBALANCES:

- **Estrogen Dominance:** This is when estrogen overshadows other hormones, which can cause changes in sleep patterns, increased body fat, increased appetite, headaches, higher perceived stress, mood swings, and slowed metabolism.
- **Polycystic Ovarian Syndrome (PCOS):** PCOS is a bit of a hormone hurricane in itself. It causes a disruption in ovulation, low progesterone, high testosterone, and often high insulin, which can all lead to infertility, weight gain, a higher risk for diabetes and infertility, belly fat, facial hair, hair loss, depression, irregular cycles, and acne.
- **Disorder of Testosterone Production:** Women with high stress often find themselves with very low levels of testosterone due to plummeting levels of

cortisol, which can lead to loss of drive, insomnia, weight gain, muscle loss, an inability to manage stress, skin problems, sexual issues, lack of creativity, and a loss of excitement for new things.

- **Hypothyroidism:** Low thyroid due to ongoing high stress affects the production of progesterone and ultimately causes estrogen dominance. It can lead to slowed metabolism, weight gain, skin problems, fuzzy brain, inflammation, high cholesterol, brittle hair and nails, head hair loss, and digestive issues.
- **Infertility:** Lack of ovulation can lead to insufficient progesterone and irregular cycles or heavy bleeding.
- **Anovulation:** This is when no ovulation or intermittent ovulation occurs. It can lead to imbalance in estrogen or progesterone, depression, anxiety, period problems, tender breasts, PMS, menopausal symptoms, and sleep issues.
- **Adrenal Fatigue:** Low levels of cortisol (after months or years of high cortisol) lead to low-functioning adrenals, which can cause exhaustion, muscle aches and pains, anxiety, depression, insomnia or wakefulness, brain fog, weight gain, and low moods.

FEMALE HORMONES

As you know by now, the specific hormones that make up the sex-hormone group are estrogen, progesterone, and testosterone. I would like to highlight each one so you might be able to see what exactly each of them does in your body and how a simple imbalance in any one can lead to a full-blown hormone hurricane.

Estrogen

Estrogen has more than 400 functions in the female body. You might even call estrogen *the mother* of all hormones. (I'm sorry, I couldn't help myself.) In all seriousness, though, I often refer to estrogen as the "nice" hormone, because when this hormone is low, women do not feel very nice. They often say they are biting people's heads off, not wanting to be social, feeling overwhelmed, and often feeling downright mean. This hormone is vital for balance. It does such things as increase our metabolic rate, regulate body temperature, maintain muscle, and improve sleep. The following are many of the things this hardworking hormone does for us:

- Increases metabolic rate

- Improves insulin sensitivity

- Regulates body temperature

- Helps maintain muscle

- Improves sleep

- Maintains memory, concentration, and word retrieval

- Regulates external body temperature

- Increases energy and vitality

- Improves blood flow and dilates small arteries

- Prevents dementia/Alzheimer's

- Maintains collagen and elasticity of the skin

- Decreases lipoprotein(a)

- Acts as a natural calcium channel blocker to keep arteries open

- Helps maintain bone density

- Helps prevent diabetes and colon cancer

- Decreases arterial plaque

- Increases moisture in the skin

- Reduces overall risk of heart disease by 40 percent

- Improves mood and concentration

- Reduces inflammation

- Helps prevent wrinkles

- Prevents macular degeneration and cataracts while protecting vision

- Prevents tooth loss and gum disease

- Stimulates the production of neurotransmitters in the brain (such as serotonin), reducing depression, anxiety, and pain

Precisely the right amount of estrogen does great things for our bodies, but many women have an excess of estrogen because they are losing progesterone due to age and stress. (You only make progesterone with ovulation, and stress reduces ovulation.) Progesterone levels are often reduced well before menopause. But estrogen and progesterone are meant to work together in a particular ratio, and when there is an imbalance, symptoms will appear that are not often diagnosed as estrogen dominance and get overlooked or dismissed as normal. While this may be common, it is not optimal.

Estrogen dominance can cause any of the following symptoms:

- Depression

- Rage and irritability

- Bloating, swelling, and water retention

- Panic attacks or anxiety

- Heavy periods

- Uterine fibroids

- Irregular uterine bleeding

- Heavy uterine bleeding

- Breast tenderness

- Hypothyroidism

- Fatigue or exhaustion

- Weight gain

- Cravings and increased appetite

- Uterine cancer, breast cancer, autoimmune disorders

Estrogen dominance is caused by a variety of factors, including (perhaps obviously) taking too much estrogen or using estrogen only. Some of the things that lead to estrogen dominance are birth control pills, vaginal rings, the use of synthetic progestins (which reduces your body's own progesterone levels), and environmental estrogens like plastics, toxins, and chemicals.

Progesterone

Symptoms of progesterone loss have patients frequently banging down our office doors. And I'm not talking metaphorically. When progesterone levels are low, women often feel as though they are losing their minds.

Antidepressants are often used for women with progesterone deficiency due to depression and anxiety, but antidepressants and antianxiety meds further reduce progesterone levels in the body while stripping the body of B vitamins and magnesium, which can make moods and anxiety even worse.

Progesterone is a hormone high up on the hormone manufacturing chain. As a result, a loss of progesterone can lead to a secondary loss of many other hormones in the hormone manufacturing cycle (as shown in the following figure).

The Female Hormone Cycle

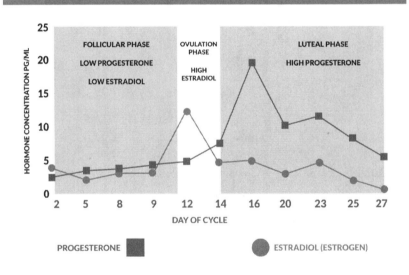

Figure 3.2: Graph of the Female Hormone Cycle

Beyond regulating your mood, one of the most important roles of progesterone is to protect the breasts. Without it, women are at a significantly increased risk for breast cancer. Increased sugar intake or foods that turn into sugar (like flour or starches) lead to lower levels of progesterone. Low levels of vitamin A, B6, vitamin C, and zinc can also lead to plummeting levels of progesterone, which can, in turn, trigger mental issues.

Low progesterone levels can cause the following symptoms:

- Anxiety and depression

- Negativity and irritability

- Heart racing, palpitations, or arrhythmias

- Irritability, rage, and irrational moods—also known as Jekyll and Hyde Syndrome

- Weight gain

- Tender, swollen breasts

- Increased inflammation and pain

- Insomnia

- Heavy or irregular bleeding

- Heightened PMS

- Early menopause symptoms

PROGESTERONE VS. SYNTHETIC PROGESTINS

Synthetic progesterone is called *progestin*, and you'd be forgiven for thinking that it's a surefire way to treat low levels of natural progesterone. The truth is much more complicated. Progestins do not reproduce the same actions of natural progesterone. In fact, when used in contraceptive or hormone therapy, they reduce the body's natural progesterone production (making everything worse).

For example, contraceptives stay in the body longer, occupying the receptor site of progesterone, often for months (which is why women who go off the pill often do not have regular periods or feel just as bad off birth control as they did on it). Progestins do protect against uterine cancer, but they provide no benefit to the breasts. They also counteract the positive effects of estrogen on serotonin, making depression, anxiety, and chronic pain worse. The following is a list of effects progestins have on the body:

- Increase appetite

- Increase weight gain and water retention

- Increase depression and anxiety

- Decrease energy and stamina

- Reduce sex drive and vitality

- Cause headaches

- Increase breast tenderness

- Cause acne, oily, and aging skin

- Increase hair loss

- Increase nausea

- Increase insomnia

- Increase "estrogen dominance"

Testosterone

Last but not least, the sex hormone most women are surprised to hear they need to stay in balance is testosterone. That's right; it's not just for men anymore. (Not that it ever was.) Women low in testosterone will often tell me they feel like they have lost their edge. They feel emotionally and physically weak. And most importantly for the brilliant women I see, they feel like they can't manage their stress anymore. They feel weak and frazzled, like they are constantly overreacting in stressful situations.

Another tragic victim of low testosterone is a woman's libido. These women find that they could care less about sex and then feel guilty for not having a sex drive or trying to please their man. The reality that we need to acknowledge here is that sex makes women feel great. If women have enough testosterone to even have a drive and subsequently have good, satisfying sex, they will feel happier, sexier, healthier, younger, and more hormonally balanced. Following are some of the symptoms of low testosterone:

- Dry skin, excessive wrinkling

- Fatigue, exhaustion

- Compromised memory and focus

- Confusion

- Insomnia

- Pale skin

- Dry eyes

- Fat gain in the belly and on the chest

- Loss of sex drive and reduced ability to have an orgasm

- Infertility

- Decreased strength and loss of muscle mass

- Hair loss; brittle hair and nails

- Overreacting to stress

- Feeling sad or not excited about life or future plans

- Feeling stressed or overwhelmed

As bad as low testosterone can be, high testosterone can be even worse. Because while low testosterone can leave a woman feeling sluggish and asexual, elevated levels can make you feel, frankly... a bit too *masculine*. Fortunately, the signs of elevated testosterone are usually more apparent in women than most hormonal imbalances and commonly present alongside a larger issue such as PCOS or metabolic syndrome. As such, these issues often get diagnosed and treated before they get out of hand. However, it is still worth looking out for the symptoms.

Polycystic ovarian syndrome has been closely correlated with high stress and adrenal dysfunction. Some of the symptoms of PCOS and elevated high testosterone that could be associated with high insulin include:

- Weight gain

- Oily skin

- Acne

- Facial hair

- Rage, irritability, depression, mood swings

- High insulin (fat storage hormone)

It's important to remember, though, that testosterone has a wealth of benefits for women when it's expressed at the proper level. Besides helping women enjoy a more fulfilling sex life, testosterone can help women ward off heart disease (which is the number one killer of women) and breast cancer. An intriguing report in the *Journal of Women's Health* examined the hypothesis that testosterone deficiency is a key factor in heart disease in aging women or women who have had a hysterectomy with ovaries removed at an earlier age. Women who had this procedure prior to menopause have a threefold increase in cardiovascular disease compared to women who have not had this surgery. The study then ultimately showed that menopausal women using testosterone get protective benefits to the heart at any age.[9]

Renowned researcher in the area of female sexuality, Dr. Susan Davis, in the *Journal of Clinical Endocrinology and Metabolism*, says that testosterone therapy in women produced a direct, sustained improvement in sex drive, arousal, the ability to climax efficiently, and the frequency of sexual fantasies[10] (all of which are important for women at any age). Please do not forget that healthy, satisfying sex is a fantastic antiaging therapy and is amazing for your mood, brain, and hormone balance.

Testosterone has many benefits besides sex, which include the following:

- Preserving muscle

- Mental focus and concentration

- Assisting with managing everyday stress

- Feeling excited about life

- Enhancing and preserving personal creativity and vitality

9   Dennis A. Davey, "Androgens in Women before and after the Menopause and Post Bilateral Oophorectomy: Clinical Effects and Indications for Testosterone Therapy," *Women's Health* 8, no. 4 (2012), doi: 10.2217/WHE.12.27.

10 Susan Davis, "Androgen Replacement in Women: A Commentary," The Journal of Clinical Endocrinology & Metabolism 84, no. 6 (1999), doi: 10.1010/jcem.84.6.5802.

- Building bones and preventing bone loss

- Strength, stamina, and coordination

- Enhancing mood and significantly reducing anxiety

- Enhancing skin elasticity and lubrication, delaying the effects of aging on the skin

- Increasing blood flow and circulation to the heart

- Improving sagging cheeks and thin lips

- Treating migraines

- Protecting the breasts

- Preventing dry, breaking, and thinning hair

- Improving self-esteem

- Treating low or lost sex drive and interest in sexual activity

- Making you feel young again

If you think you may have some type of hormone imbalance or deficiency that may be connected to stress in some way, it is time to consider scheduling an appointment with your doctor for testing and treatment. When you walk into your medical practitioner's office, you will often get a hormone lab slip for routine blood work such as a CBC (complete blood count) or serum chemistry tests to get an overall snapshot of what is happening in your body. However, few practitioners will order a comprehensive panel of lifesaving hormone levels such as DHEA, progesterone, estrogen, and testosterone levels. Unfortunately, most doctors and practitioners today have no clue that a youthful balance of hormones—the body's vital chemical messengers—are essential to your overall emotional, physical, and mental well-being.

If your sex hormones, stress hormones, or thyroid hormones are depleted, you will most likely be suffering from many side effects and symptoms that are often written off and ignored as stress or aging. But given the numerous studies that show the many associations between failing hormone levels and age-related disorders such as Alzheimer's and heart disease, there should be no doubt that testing for these specific failing hormone levels at any age should be part of a yearly checkup and prevention program. Wouldn't it make more sense to find the imbalance or deficiency and then fix it? Maybe one day we'll learn. Until then, it's up to you to take the initiative in your health care and request the tests and treatments necessary to keep your body and mind in brilliant shape.

WHAT IS THE BEST WAY TO TEST YOUR HORMONES?

There are three options for testing hormones: blood, urine, and saliva. Each method has pros and cons, and each one provides unique information. This should be taken into consideration when deciding which test is best for you. At my office, we use serum (blood) testing for most hormone imbalances, as I have found this to be the easiest, clearest, most efficient method of identifying a hormone imbalance. Blood tests directly correlate with symptoms and are usually covered by insurance companies.

Blood Testing (Serum)

Most hormone specialists today endorse hormone testing, and the simplest way to test hormones is through a blood test. The assays used in serum testing are precise and are not influenced radically by the hormones that are taken orally, sublingually, or topically, like the assays in saliva testing are. Blood serum testing is a tried-and-true way to check hormones and is regarded by many to be an excellent approach, as it is accurate, convenient, assessable, and covered by most insurance companies.

I have tested hormones for over 27 years using serum testing, and it consistently provides results in line with my patients' (both women and men) symptoms, supplying an excellent guide for me to treat them. The Centers for Disease Control and Prevention (CDC) has even launched a program to check the accuracy and reliability of blood testing. The CDC makes the names of the lab tests that have passed the performance criteria available on its website (www.cdc.gov), and hormone testing is among the tests listed there that have been approved for accuracy.

The important complication to keep in mind with serum testing in women, though, is to make sure the levels are tested in the second half of the woman's cycle, ideally between days 18 and 24 of her monthly cycle (counting day one of bleeding as day one of the cycle). For a woman who has had a hysterectomy but still has her ovaries, we recommend two samples, two weeks apart, to see if progesterone and estrogen are cycling (because there is no period to go by for testing in the right phase). Because women are ideally supposed to make 80 percent of their progesterone after day 14 of the cycle, it is best to test during this time for the cycling and changing hormones of estrogen and progesterone.

I typically order a full hormone panel (thyroid, ovaries, and adrenals) at the first visit for women in menopause. If they are not in menopause and in the right phase of their cycle or have had a hysterectomy and the ovaries are still intact, we repeat only the estrogen and progesterone levels again in two weeks to see if cycling is occurring. All other women can have a single sample test according to the cycle (second half) or in menopause (including women with a hysterectomy and ovaries removed) anytime.

The 24-Hour Urinary Panel

The 24-hour urinary hormone panel can test more of the daily fluctuations in hormone levels. It also tests the fractionated estrogens (estrone, estradiol, and estriol) and provides additional information such as the levels of 2:16 hydroxyestrone ratio and 2-Methoxyestradiol (suspected to have anticancer qualities). However, this test is more expensive than blood or saliva tests and needs to be done in the home. This test also has some limitations in that it only measures the hormones the body is excreting in the urine. While this information is often useful, it does not always correlate with the action of the hormones in the blood or at the tissue level.

Saliva Testing

Saliva testing is also done in the home. It looks mostly at free hormone levels and allows the practitioner to see the charting of the hormones throughout the month (taking saliva samples throughout the cycle to see the rhythm of hormones or throughout the day to see the rhythm of cortisol throughout a 24-hour period).

The results of saliva testing, however, are not always accurate. Hormones are found in much lower concentrations in the saliva than in the blood, and this makes test-to-test comparisons less consistent and harder to report. In addition, women who are taking bioidentical hormones will show very high levels in the saliva, which some labs account for in their reference range, but the range is so broad that it is difficult to interpret accurately. Additionally, saliva tests only the free hormones, and, in the case of cortisol, the free cortisol is only 1 percent of the total cortisol in the body.

As you can see, there are pros and cons with each method of testing. But if you are starting the journey of taming your personal hormone hurricane, I advise you to brave the needle and go with the blood test. With serum blood testing we use the most sensitive assays, methods, and laboratory equipment for hormone testing currently available. Do keep in mind, though, that there is quite a bit of variability between commercial laboratories. Labs utilize different methods, and some of these methods, unfortunately, have less accuracy and a greater variability, which I believe compromise the results.

WHEN TO TEST YOUR HORMONES

So now that you are familiar with the tests, when should you plan your doctor's appointment to get them done? Well, if you are still cycling with regular periods, testing should be done after ovulation, so sometime between days 16 and 24 of the cycle (16 days after the first day of your period). If you have had a hysterectomy with one or more ovaries left in place *and* you are not menopausal in age, then testing at two different times, two weeks apart, is best. This will show if you are still cycling or not. If you are menopausal with no period or have had a hysterectomy with both ovaries removed, testing can be done at any time of the month. If you have PMS or significant problems at certain times of the month, such as migraines, dizziness, seizures, depression, or anxiety, try to test at that particular time of the cycle.

Hormone Tests Needed for Evaluating an Imbalance

It is important to get the correct tests to determine if your hormones are balanced. I recommend the following panel:

- Estradiol (estrogen)

- Progesterone

- Free and total testosterone

- DHEA-S

- Thyroid panel—TSH, free T4, free T3 (also possible addition of thyroid antibodies and reverse T3 levels)

- Cortisol (morning and late afternoon reading is best)

- Pregnenolone

INTERPRETING THE RESULTS:

I recommend that you get your testing done between days 18 and 21 of your cycle. The following levels are considered ideal and should help you gauge your results:

- Estradiol levels should be within 80–200 in the second half of the monthly cycle (after day 14 of the cycle)

- Progesterone levels should be above 5

- Testosterone levels should be above 40 and preferably around 60 (depending on the symptoms, goals, and side effects)

- DHEA-S should be around 200

- Pregnenolone should be a minimum of 120

Women who have had hysterectomies and have ovaries still intact should have at least one of the two samples that were drawn with the same results as a cycling woman:

- Estradiol levels should be within 80–200 in the cycling phase of the cycle

- Progesterone levels should be above 5

- Testosterone levels should be above 40 and preferably around 60 (depending on the symptoms/goals/side effects)

- DHEA-S should be around 200

- Pregnenolone should be a minimum of 120

Postmenopausal women on hormone therapy (bioidentical) *and* women who have had hysterectomies with ovaries removed can expect slightly different readings.

- Estradiol levels should be within 50–150 (if taking estradiol)

- Progesterone levels should be between 2–10 (if taking progesterone)

- Testosterone levels should be above 40 and preferably around 60 (if using Testosterone)

- DHEA-S should be above 100 and preferably between 100–300

- Pregnenolone should be a minimum of 120 or higher if symptomatic

WHAT HORMONE SPECIALISTS ARE LOOKING FOR

Beyond the mere numbers, hormone imbalance has many hallmarks that most hormone specialists keep an eye out for. Lab tests show if hormones are below normal and whether they match up with the symptoms a woman is experiencing. It is critical that the lab reports are closely correlated with a woman's symptoms.

Ideally, it's best to test hormones on a regular basis so you have lots of data to compare. Test when you feel amazing, with no symptoms, and also when you feel like crap, suffering through the side effects of hormonal changes. This helps to not only define abnormal imbalances, deficiencies, or excess hormone levels but also defines what normal and ideal looks like for any particular woman. Every single woman is different and has a unique balance and range that is best for them. That's why the best treatment for women is testing every 90 days to ensure that the levels are normal and optimal *for them*. Stress can affect the production and balance of nearly every hormone, so periodic testing as stressful situations arise help women stay on top of plummeting levels or imbalances that lead to a myriad of symptoms.

If any medical practitioner or doctor tells you that hormone levels cannot be tested due to fluctuations, please do not listen to this. This is old, outdated nonsense, and the information that testing can give hormone experts is invaluable in helping women of all ages completely turn around and eliminate the ongoing, nagging, and awful symptoms of hormone imbalance. It really works.

TREATING HORMONE IMBALANCES WITH BIOIDENTICAL HORMONES

Once testing is completed, the next step is to determine where the imbalance is and exactly how to treat it. Bioidentical hormones are plant based and replicated from your own hormones, and can be used to correct deficiencies, excesses, and true imbalances in all hormone levels. The signs and symptoms of hormone imbalance can include fatigue, depression, hair loss, headaches, heavy periods, weight gain, muscle atrophy, low energy levels, insomnia, mood swings, hot flashes, night sweats, loss of sex drive, and anxiety. Bioidentical hormone replacement therapy (BHRT) may not be necessary but can be used effectively to completely resolve hormone imbalance side effects and promote better aging and zest for life. Below are some of the specific hormones that can be tested and what they do.

Progesterone

Progesterone can be compounded in the pharmacy or prescribed as Prometrium, which is commercially available at all pharmacies and is plant based and bioidentical. I typically will use a progesterone cream, however, if a woman has cystic breasts, depression, mood problems, or anxiety, as this seems to work best for these particular problems.

Progesterone is nearly always used at bedtime, as it has a calming effect and helps induce sleep. If a woman has daytime anxiety or advanced low-functioning adrenals (low or high cortisol), progesterone can be used in smaller dosages (30–50mg) two to three times per day when applied to the skin. It can also be used directly on the breasts for treating cystic or painful breasts, which works amazingly well.

Progesterone is safe to use and will often calm the heart racing or palpitations women have with stress. I always prescribe progesterone (bioidentical) with a birth control pill, as I believe it protects against estrogen dominance, which leads to breast problems, weight gain, and mood disorders. Progesterone is also sold over the counter in small dosages of 20–30mg in a cream form.

Estrogen

Estrogen can be administered in the form of a pill, a sublingual lozenge, a patch, a vaginal cream or insert (for vaginal dryness), or a topical cream. This hormone often needs replacing during menopause and not as often when a woman is still menstruating. During menopause, it helps to alleviate the ongoing symptoms of insomnia, blood sugar instability, weight gain, foggy memory, and other aging effects. In menopause, dosages vary from 0.25 mg to 2 mg daily. This hormone can be used once or twice daily and can be prescribed commercially as estradiol in a pill or patch or can be compounded with plant-based bioidentical hormones in any dose or method of administration desired.

It is the hormone most likely to be too dominant in women who are menstruating and under a great deal of stress. Estrogen, when dominant, should be buffered with progesterone and testosterone to get the right balance. We often will use a DIM supplement and zinc or saw palmetto to effectively speed up the metabolization of estrogen that is not needed. The liver can be supported with supplements like milk thistle or our proprietary supplement we carry called Liver C, which is extremely effective in supporting the liver and enhancing the disposal of excess estrogen in the body.

Testosterone

Testosterone should only be prescribed in a bioidentical form and is only available in this form from a compounding pharmacy. It is most often prescribed as a cream or vaginal insert. A pill form is available but not suggested, as it is not advised to have testosterone make its first pass of the body through the liver. The cream can be used on the body (in a measured amount) and also used in the vaginal or labial area (mucous membrane) for more enhanced absorption. It is most effective in an implantable pellet for under the skin.

Testosterone dosing is typically 0.5–6mg daily, depending on the situation, symptoms, side effects, and age. In younger women, DHEA supplements can be used to help boost testosterone levels, which can be very effective. Testosterone can be used in women on hormonal contraceptives, antidepressants, or high blood pressure medications, which can often cause low levels of testosterone. Ongoing stress also plummets testosterone, leaving a woman feeling as if she can't manage stress, which of course makes the stress worse.

DHEA

DHEA can be taken as a capsule or tablet and is sold over the counter, or it can be prescribed and made into a cream, vaginal insert (good for lubrication, atrophy, and incontinence), or sublingual lozenge, tablet, or pill at a compounding pharmacy. The typical dosage of DHEA is 5–50mg, depending on the age, blood level, and symptoms of the individual. Typically, women very low in DHEA with some sort of autoimmune problem will use higher dosages and work up to these levels. Younger, highly stressed women typically use the lower doses to start with, and menopausal women will often simply use 25 mg daily to support the adrenals and their testosterone levels.

Hormone Pellet Therapy

This is by far my most favorite way to administer hormones at any age. Seriously, I love this method, and you will too: bioidentical hormone supplementation. How it works is that pellets are fused with plant-based hormones that are customized to the dose you need and about the size of a puffed-up piece of rice. Then, this pellet is implanted in the fatty tissue of the upper buttocks (under the skin). The pellets for women work continuously for up to five months—just implant 'em and forget 'em. They release according to heart rate and cardiac output, so when you are exercising, stressed, having sex, or doing anything that raises your heart rate, you release more of the hormone via the pellet directly into your body's circulatory system. And when you are resting, sleeping, or taking it easy and your heart rate is lower, you release less.

This is in line with how the body would naturally release hormones. I like this method for women who need a boost in testosterone and want instant action and fewer side effects. The pellets begin releasing to optimal levels within 72 hours of implantation and are highly effective for overachieving women today who need the support and have documented low testosterone levels. This approach is also versatile in that we can use estradiol, progesterone, and testosterone in a pellet form. In many younger women who are on the pill or antidepressants, have migraine headaches or PMS, or suffer a lack of sex drive, we can use a testosterone pellet alone. We also use it consistently in menopausal women, as it protects against dementia, breast cancer, and heart disease.

All hormone levels with the pellets are tested with each insertion of the hormones, which allows us to use smaller dosages with better results and the least amount of side effects. Do your due diligence before opting for this therapy because the dosage of the pellet therapy is terribly important, and not all medical providers offering pellet therapy have a deep understanding of proper dosing. I feel strongly that this is a key component to getting hormonally balanced safely and effectively.

ADDITIONAL TREATMENT OPTIONS FOR HORMONAL BALANCE

In some cases, bioidentical hormones may not be necessary; diet, lifestyle, and environmental factors have a serious impact on hormone balance and must be looked at as part of the big picture. I have repeatedly told my patients that diet is at least 50 percent of their recovery, and without the implementation of a balanced lifestyle and diet, they will likely not achieve full recovery of their ongoing symptoms.

Carbs and Healthy Fats

If you would consider giving up carbs (not veggies but other starchy carbs) and substitute them for good fats, your hormones would thank you. That's right, I'm telling you to eat fat for your health. Well, it's actually more complex than that, but still—YAY! All hormones come from fat, so an unhealthy fat diet or a low-fat diet can both make a hormone imbalance worse. Your body needs various types of fats to create hormones and to help keep inflammation down, which further supports good hormone balance.

Unhealthy starchy-sugary-carbohydrate foods and drinks have the opposite effect. They cause inflammation and fatigue and mess with the balance of your hormones. So if you want to go about revamping your diet to fix your hormones, here are a few simple first steps you can take.

Immediately eliminate the unhealthy vegetable oils, such as safflower, sunflower, corn, cottonseed, peanut, canola, and soybean, and instead start consuming more coconut oil. You should also consume nuts, seeds, avocados, salmon, and focus on more omega-3 fats and fewer omega-6 fats. (Omega-3 fats help protect the brain and are anti-inflammatory.) Consider the supplement evening primrose oil, which helps balance omega-3 and 6 and also provides support for hormone balance.

Life Coaches, Journaling, and Meditation

This is such an important step in balancing your hormones and your life, but it's rarely easy. To help get your emotions in balance, you may want to hire a life coach or start journaling your feelings. Getting your head in the right spot will take you miles into a healthy hormonal balance. Do not ignore this step, as it is paramount to getting you 100 percent balanced and on the right track to managing your daily stress and where your brain goes because of it.

Many practitioners for emotional well-being believe that the emotion of fear causes disruption in the sex organs, which can lead to a hormone imbalance. This can also lead to PCOS and infertility, erratic cycles, and estrogen dominance. That's why it's best to be mindful and never let yourself stagnate in a place of fear.

Similar problems arise with the emotions of impatience, the inability to forgive, and frustration, which can lead to serious issues with the liver, where your hormones are excreted, leading to a potential imbalance. The emotions of worry and anxiety can cause issues with your insulin levels, which affect all hormones and lead to weight gain in the belly. Practicing 5 to 30 minutes of guided or silent meditation daily may be the only time you have to quiet your precious brain and nervous system. This practice can also make it much easier for you to break out of the cycles of these emotions and free yourself from their physical effects. You need a daily reboot for your emotional and mental well-being. Your emotions and hormones are closely connected, so balancing one will optimally support the other. For maximum benefit, make meditation part of your daily routine. You may also want to consider regular massage and acupuncture as adjuncts for support.

Supplementation

In addition to the self-care above, supplements will work wonders toward restoring balance and helping you feel better. Some of my favorites are the following:

VITAMIN D

This fat-soluble vitamin acts like a hormone inside the body and is vital for keeping inflammation down. Plus, it's a natural mood improver and will give you energy and better brain function with a good dose of immunity against the flu and other illnesses. Most women need 3,000–5,000 units of vitamin D taken daily with food—and preferably food high in healthy fats for the best absorption.

PROBIOTICS

To repair the gut and to optimize the absorption of nutrients in your diet, consider taking this supplement daily. Probiotics are healthy bacteria that can improve the production and regulation of hormones in your body. Optimally, the dose should be more than 20 billion CFU.

BRAIN CHEMICAL SUPPORT

Amino acids are direct precursors to your brain chemicals and are necessary for support, as they directly interact with hormones in the body. Supporting serotonin, dopamine, norepinephrine, GABA, and endorphins will help you get rid of nagging moods, anxiety, and concentration issues and will positively support the hormone changes made. Adding lean, healthy organic proteins in your diet will also support these amino acids.

Beware of Medications That Ransack Your Hormones

Medications prescribed today for symptom or medical issues often change or, at times, even create a hormone deficiency. These can lead to serious side effects like loss of sex drive, fatigue, appetite changes, altered sleep patterns, or depression. Corticosteroids (prednisone), stimulants (drugs prescribed for attention deficit disorder), statins (drugs prescribed to regulate cholesterol), dopamine agonists, blood pressure medications, hormonal birth control, and antidepressants can all change hormone levels and create a terrible imbalance. If you must use these medications, make sure you are also keeping track of your levels and using bioidentical hormones to balance your hormones and reduce side effects.

Essential Oils for Hormone Balance

Today, more and more women are experiencing the amazing effects of essential oils. These can not only help eliminate toxins in the body but can provide balance to women suffering from estrogen overload. I recommend using the following:

THYME

Thyme increases progesterone production and helps to treat hormone imbalances like estrogen dominance. Use 3–5 drops in bath water or rub into coconut oil and apply to your abdomen.

CLARY SAGE

Clary sage helps balance estrogen levels because it contains natural phytoestrogens. It can be used to help support the menstrual cycle, relieve PMS symptoms, and treat infertility and PCOS. It also helps relieve anxiety and depression. Rubbing two to three drops above the eyebrow one to three times daily can be quite effective for relief. (See Appendix C.)

FENNEL

Fennel reduces inflammation, boosts metabolism, promotes sleep, and heals gut problems. Consider mixing 5–7 drops in coconut oil rubbed on your gut or pelvic area.

LAVENDER

Lavender promotes emotional balance, as it helps treat anxiety, depression, moodiness, and stress. Mix 5–7 drops in coconut oil and rub it on the back of your neck or wrists. It can be used in baths or at bedtime or whenever you need some extra relief.

SANDALWOOD

Sandalwood can be used to increase your sex drive, reduce stress, and promote relaxation (especially when you are keyed up at the end of the work day and don't want to take it out on your loved ones). Mix 3–5 drops in coconut oil and apply to your wrists or feet. You can also inhale it before applying it.

Avoiding Toxic Chemical Exposure

It sounds strange, but everyday items you use and consume may be contributing to your hormonal upheaval. Conventional body care products that are made with harmful chemicals, including DEA, parabens, sodium lauryl sulfate, or propylene glycol, can increase the problem of estrogen dominance. These chemicals are estrogen mimickers in the body and are a surefire way of creating an imbalance.

Natural products like coconut oil, castor oil, or shea butter are optimal for the skin and do not contain harmful chemicals. I often send my patients to the Environmental Working Group (EWG) website to find out what products are harmful and what products are best for the skin and contain no toxins (www.ewg.org). This site contains over 75,000 products that have been evaluated based on their hidden toxins and is a great resource for women like you who are looking to take control of their hormones.

FAST-TRACK PLAN FOR HORMONE BALANCE

I know that I've just given you a lot of information, and you may be wondering where to begin with all of it. I also know how important it is not to be overwhelmed with all of this, so below are my suggestions for how to fast track your hormones into balance and achieve the most efficient results.

- Get tested at the right time of your cycle or according to the suggestions in this chapter (see Appendix F for testing options).

- Immediately change your diet to eating fewer sugary and starchy carbohydrates, and incorporating good fats into each day. (Try no sugar or flour products for 14 days; I guarantee, once the cravings fade you will feel infinitely better.)

- Include lots of coconut oil, oily fish, nuts, seeds, and chia in your diet.

- Start eating leafy greens and lots of them, with one to two fruits per day (low sugar like apples).

- Eat only lean proteins (organic is best).

- Add DIM supplement to enhance estrogen metabolism (see Appendix B).

- Go to bed early in order to get up early and still get a minimum of seven hours of sleep. If you are not sleeping, start a sleep supplement or the stress supplements suggested in Appendix D to support the optimal cortisol rhythm. Try this for 14 days and make sure you are staying asleep.

- Start bioidentical hormones once testing is available to correct deficiencies or imbalances.

- Start using natural cleaning products and less plastic in the home. Switch to chemical-free soaps and shampoos.

- Start a mindful meditation practice, or go to sleep at night listening to meditations.

- Stop the negative language, and make your mantra, "I am healthy and balanced and love my life" (even if you don't believe it yet).

- Stop overeating, and begin increasing the number of hours per day that you are fasting. Attempt to get to 13 hours minimum of daily fasting (i.e., stop eating at 8 p.m. and do not eat again until 9 a.m.) or more if possible. This will reduce the burden of your body having to ramp up its energy stores to digest the food you are constantly eating. This tip alone will increase your energy and reduce your body fat.

- Start exercising daily (preferably outside) for a minimum of 15 minutes. Work up to a type of exercise that is high-intensity intervals (HIIT). This not only will make you feel great, but it will also carve off the fat, support your stress glands, and help you manufacture more human growth hormone, which will slow aging and start giving you energy and stamina.

- Start supplementing with vitamin B complex, magnesium, zinc, and vitamin D3 (1,000 units for each 25–50 pounds of body weight).

- Consider a mood support supplement of amino acids that will support the neuro brain chemicals that are often low due to fluctuating levels of hormones (see Appendix C). This allows women to achieve emotional balance more timely.

Hormone Hurricane Success Story

Gina arrived in my office feeling totally defeated. She had seen her gynecologist in the previous year with the exact same problems she was seeing me for: fatigue, intermittent depression, inability to turn off her brain at night, exhaustion, feeling overwhelmed, a lack of concentration and focus in school, and missed periods. In the past, these issues had mostly been ignored. She was prescribed birth control and an antianxiety medication to help her sleep and take the edge off. Ultimately, though, she kept being told to just relax and stop stressing.

Gina started the antianxiety and birth control pills and continued her rather full life of taking care of her three kids while going to aesthetician school and trying her best to keep it all together. She desperately wanted to feel better, but after six months of using the birth control and antianxiety medication, she felt even worse. She felt more depressed than before, and her memory was getting to the point that her instructors were wondering if she could hold it together for graduation. She was given no guidance on diet, stress reduction, or supplements, and she was never offered any form of hormone testing.

I told her we were going to change that. She was tested in my office and found to have *zero* progesterone (which was causing her intermittent depression, irregular cycles, and anxiety). She also had rock-bottom testosterone levels (leading to no drive or endurance, foggy thinking, and feeling overwhelmed) and low cortisol in the morning (when it is supposed to be high for energy and focus) and high cortisol at night (when it is supposed to be low so you can turn off your brain and go to sleep). To make matters worse, she was also deficient in most of the vitamins we all need in our daily life—vitamin D, B12, DHEA (stress), and ferritin (iron storage).

As we reviewed her labs and made a plan for recovery, we were quickly able to zero in on a few simple changes she could make in her life and medical regimen.

Her game plan included the following:

- Immediately correcting the nutrient deficiencies with natural vitamins and starting a supplementation plan to keep them in the optimal ranges

- Starting on a gluten-, sugar-, and starch-free diet

- Receiving weekly vitamin B injections for vitality and mental support

- Getting a testosterone pellet implanted to boost her energy and help give her clarity and focus

- Correcting her progesterone levels with a prescription cream that would immediately help treat her anxiety and fix her estrogen dominant state

This plan worked better than Gina could have ever hoped. Over the course of the next 90 days, she was able to get off the antianxiety medication (which was causing amnesia and forgetfulness and is terribly addictive) and the birth control pills that were creating a further imbalance (she'd had a tubal ligation, so she did not need this for birth control anyway). She continues to see me every six months to make sure her levels are staying balanced, and she thrives in a busy aesthetician practice now while keeping all of the balls in the air with ease. Most importantly, though, every time I see her, she is smiling and happy and making sure she sticks to the basics of self-care and hormone balance so she can more easily stay in the game.

4

Thyroid Madness: The Burden of Stress on Your Metabolism . . . Rescuing This Vital Powerhouse

"Not to brag or anything . . . but I can forget what I am doing, while I am doing it!"

—*LUCILLE BALL*

In this chapter, we will explore the important role your thyroid gland plays in your day-to-day life. Take the following quiz to see if your thyroid is low.

QUIZ: IS YOUR THYROID LOW?

1. Are you overweight or accumulating more fat for no reason? Y/N
2. Do you have a history of yo-yo dieting and weight loss or gain? Y/N

3. Are you fatigued, especially in the afternoon? Y/N

4. Are you prone to cold hands and feet? Y/N

5. Does your head feel too heavy or tired? Y/N

6. Does your energy drop in the afternoon? Y/N

7. Is there a swelling of the throat area or do you have a voice-strain problem (raspy, coarse, or weak voice)? Y/N

8. Do you have constipation (bowel straining or not eliminating daily)? Y/N

9. Is the outside portion of your eyebrows thinning or gone? Y/N

10. Do you have dry skin or skin problems? Y/N

11. Do you have dark patches or rough skin on your elbows? Y/N

12. Are your muscles weak, achy, or prone to cramping? Y/N

13. Do you have vertical ridges on your nails? Y/N

14. Do your fingernails break, crack, split, or peel? Y/N

15. Is your hair falling out or thinning? Y/N

16. Are you on thyroid medication but still do not feel your best? Y/N

17. Have you been told your thyroid is normal but you have multiple symptoms of low thyroid or tested previously on the low end of "normal"? Y/N

If you answered yes to at least three of the above questions, it may be time for a full analysis of your thyroid health. If you answered yes to all 17, then the time for that was awhile ago—get yourself to a doctor, girl!

THE CONNECTION BETWEEN HIGH STRESS AND PLUMMETING THYROID HEALTH

We all deal with stress every day. Whether we're constantly running late, taking care of loved ones, facing an important work deadline, running on fumes because of little sleep, or simply trying to get through a to-do list that never ends, we are all dealing with stress on some level. But all this rushing around can be bad news for your thyroid—a delicate gland that can sense when our bodies are out of whack. While there's no definitive proof that stress causes thyroid problems, the two definitely go hand in hand, and stress often appears to be the culprit behind low thyroid output and the reason behind why we are often dragging ourselves around, exhausted and barely getting through the day. Stress may also exacerbate any existing thyroid conditions, tipping a thyroid on the edge of normal functioning into the low-functioning state.

As you learned in the first chapter (unless you're here because you took a shortcut—no judgment), in an emergency, stress can save your life. When you are faced with a threatening situation, your body recognizes the danger and pours stress hormones into your bloodstream. These hormones drive up your heart rate and blood pressure, giving you the extra boost of energy and strength you need to survive each threatening situation (even if you're just running late to a meeting).

The connection between the thyroid gland and stress lies in the fact that the thyroid gland controls how quickly your body uses energy, makes proteins, and responds to other hormones. So, if you are making demands on your body by constantly calling for stress hormones (as most busy people do), then the response from the thyroid is to attempt to keep up with the energy demands until it just can't do it anymore. Like driving a car pedal to the metal all the time—eventually it will break down. Then, all you can do is shift into the lowest possible gear and try to make it to the shop. The same thing happens to your body. If you push your thyroid too far, your body begins to feel broken down.

The HPA axis is a complex network that connects the hypothalamus, the pituitary gland, and the adrenal glands. Numerous studies have shown that stress weakens this entire process, so when the HPA axis is depressed, it can likewise downregulate the production of thyroid hormones and the thyroid's general function. In addition, research continues to show that inflammatory cytokines, which are released during stress response, can compromise the entire HPA axis, causing a reduced level of

TSH (thyroid-stimulating hormone), which ultimately lowers the production of thyroid hormones. This interaction is also why a TSH test alone is not sufficient to evaluate someone for a thyroid disorder.

An additional connection between stress and low thyroid is that stress compromises the conversion of T4 (storage thyroid) into T3 (active thyroid). Approximately 85 percent or more of the thyroid hormone made by the thyroid gland is T4, but this is an inactive form of the molecule and must be converted to active T3 before it can be used by the cells in the body. The inflammatory cytokines produced by stress not only disrupt this process, but they also interfere with your cells' ability to utilize T3 at all, which is not good.

So let's talk about the thyroid itself to give you a better understanding of what this powerful gland does and how to manage its health better. This will help you articulate what you believe might be going on in your own body at your next medical visit.

THE THYROID GLAND

The thyroid is part of the endocrine system in the body and is a two-inch, tiny butterfly-shaped gland sitting on both sides of the bottom of your neck, just below your Adam's apple. This very small gland (right and left lobe) packs a huge punch, as it plays a part in running nearly every bodily system. The thyroid's main job is to fire up the genes that keep cells doing their job in every area of your body; it gives you energy and regulates metabolism. The thyroid hormones interact with nearly everything and are responsible for the most basic functions of the brain, digestive system, and cardiac system, while also playing a role in bone metabolism, red blood cell metabolism, lipid and cholesterol metabolism, gall bladder and liver function, glucose metabolism, protein metabolism, and body temperature.

To use another vehicle metaphor, think of your thyroid as a car engine that sets the pace at which your body operates. An engine produces the required amount of energy for a car to move at a certain speed. In the same way, your thyroid gland manufactures enough thyroid hormone to prompt your cells to perform a function at a certain rate.

Just as a car can't produce energy without gas (or electricity), your thyroid needs fuel to produce thyroid hormone. This fuel is iodine. Iodine comes from your diet and is found in iodized table salt, seafood, bread, and milk. Your thyroid extracts this necessary ingredient from your bloodstream and uses it to make two kinds of thyroid hormone: thyroxine, also called T4 because it contains four iodine atoms, and triiodothyronine, called T3 because it contains three iodine atoms. T3 is made from T4 when one atom is removed—a conversion that occurs mostly outside the thyroid in organs and tissues where T3 is used the most, such as the liver, the kidneys, and the brain.

Once T4 is produced, it is stored within the thyroid's vast number of microscopic follicles. Some T3 is also produced and stored in the thyroid, though at much lower levels. When your body needs thyroid hormone, it is secreted into your bloodstream in quantities set to meet the metabolic needs of your cells. Then, the hormone easily slips into the cells in need and attaches to special receptors located in the cells' nuclei.

Your car engine produces energy to get you moving, but you still need to tell it how fast to go by stepping on the accelerator. Likewise, the thyroid also needs some direction on how "fast" it needs to go; it gets this from your pituitary gland, which is located at the base of your brain. No larger than a pea, the pituitary gland is sometimes known as the *master gland* because it controls the functions of the thyroid and the other glands that make up the endocrine system. Your pituitary gland sends messages to your thyroid gland, telling it how much thyroid hormone to make. These messages come in the form of thyroid-stimulating hormone (TSH).

TSH levels in your bloodstream rise or fall depending on whether enough thyroid hormone is produced to meet your body's needs. Higher levels of TSH prompt the thyroid to produce more thyroid hormone. Conversely, low TSH levels signal the thyroid to slow down production.

The pituitary gland gets its information in several ways. It is able to read and respond directly to the amounts of T4 circulating in the blood, but it also responds to the hypothalamus, which is a section of the brain that releases its own hormone—thyrotropin-releasing hormone (TRH). Sticking with the driving analogy, think of the hypothalamus as the foot that pushes down on the accelerator that tells the car how fast to go. Similarly, TRH from the hypothalamus stimulates TSH production in the pituitary gland. This network of communication between the hypothalamus, the pituitary gland, and the thyroid gland is referred to as the hypothalamic-pituitary-thyroid (HPT) axis and plays an integral part in many vital functions in the body.

FUNCTIONS OF THE THYROID GLAND

The thyroid is a powerhouse system. Some of its functions include regulating:

- Metabolism (how fast you burn calories)
- Digestion
- Breathing
- Heart rate
- Temperature control
- Brain development
- Growth and development
- Carbohydrate and lipid metabolism
- Central nervous system activation or sedation
- Neuro-brain chemical balance—mood, memory, cognition
- Cardiovascular system (over or understimulation depending on the amount of thyroid hormone produced)

HYPOTHYROIDISM

Hypothyroidism is the most common thyroid disorder. However, it is still wildly underdiagnosed and often not appropriately assessed by doctors and practitioners, so let's take a moment here to focus on this condition. Hypothyroidism simply refers to a low-functioning thyroid, and for many years was not a condition the medical community was looking out for. Unfortunately, today the condition is on the rise, and a medical evaluation hardly ever takes into account how stress can make hypothyroidism worse or what can be done about it. A colleague and thyroid specialist told me years ago, "It's really not a matter of if a menopausal woman will get hypothyroidism; it's a matter of when." When I first heard this, I thought she must be exaggerating, but after testing and treating women for 27 years now, I've realized the statement is pretty accurate.

But why is this happening? And why, as it seems for so many other medical issues, are women taking the brunt of the damage? Well, the fact is that many factors, such as high-intensity daily stress, unhealthy diet, sleep patterns, fluctuating and imbalanced ovarian and adrenal hormones, and nutrient deficiencies can all lead to a hypothyroid state. The sad and scary part of all this is that women often get drugs prescribed to them to help with the symptoms of low thyroid, but these same drugs compromise the thyroid's already faulty functioning, making it worse. Drugs such as statins for high cholesterol (a common problem with low thyroid) or pain medications or anti-inflammatories for body pain or fibromyalgia (another common problem with low thyroid) are classic examples. These and many other drugs downregulate or interfere with the functioning of the thyroid, eventually causing the woman to feel worse. Kind of makes you want to punch something, huh?

According to the American Thyroid Association president, Dr. Hossein Gharib, thyroid disorders are common worldwide, not only in the US. And recent reports from the World Health Organization (WHO) even estimate that thyroid disorders affect approximately 750 million people,[11]

---

11 American Thyroid Association, "World Thyroid Day Aims to Raise Awareness of Disease," May 23, 2014, https://www.thyroid.org/world-thyroid-day-aims-to-raise-awareness-of-disease/.

and up to 60 percent of these people are unaware of their condition[12] (partially due to inadequate testing and evaluations in the medical office). This means that one in eight women will develop a thyroid disorder during her lifetime. Levothyroxine, a drug used to replace the T4 thyroid in the body and used to treat hypothyroidism, is the fourth most common selling drug in the US, with 13 out of the top 50 best-selling drugs having something to do with thyroid disorders. The number of women suffering from hypothyroidism or borderline hypothyroidism (subclinical hypothyroidism) continues to rise yearly and is especially prevalent at the onset of increased stress, perimenopause, and menopause.

SYMPTOMS OF HYPOTHYROIDISM

Hypothyroidism has some hallmark symptoms when it is low. These include the following

• Fatigue

• Weight gain or inability to lose weight

• Afternoon exhaustion (hitting a wall)

• Hair loss or dry, coarse hair (fuzzy hair)

• Brittle, splitting fingernails

• Irritable bowel symptoms, cramping, and gut problems

• Constipation

• Dry skin, skin problems, or loss of color

• Cold intolerance

• Weakness

• Brain fog—forgetfulness, lack of focus, memory loss

12 American Thyroid Association, "General Information/Press Room," accessed October 25, 2018, https://www.thyroid.org/media-main/press-room/.

- Muscle cramps and frequent muscle aches
- Sore feet (especially when you get out of bed in the morning)
- Dry, cracked heels or elbows
- Abnormal, heavy or irregular menstrual cycles
- Decreased sex drive
- Depression, irritability, sadness, and loss of zest for life
- Slow movements and thoughts
- Pain, numbness, and tingling sensation in the hands and fingers (such as carpal tunnel syndrome)
- Infertility
- Frequent infections
- Cold backside
- Fibromyalgia
- Insomnia
- Low body temperature

Long-Term Problems with an Untreated Thyroid

Many women are hesitant to treat low thyroid or even borderline low thyroid, even with the presence of many of the symptoms that point to hypothyroidism. The problem with this is that untreated low thyroid can snowball into more long-term complications, such as a low-pitched voice, an enlarged thyroid gland, chronic inflammation, high cholesterol, severe insomnia, gynecological issues with bleeding, and low sex drive. In severe cases, it can also lead to heart disease, hair loss, sleep apnea, and infertility. I mean, are you seeing all these symptoms? It's not worth ignoring this stuff. Ultimately, it is important to know the big picture when electing not to treat an imbalance, naturally or with medication.

TESTING THYROID HORMONES

Following is a list of thyroid hormone levels often tested to evaluate where each woman should optimally be. These tests should be ordered each time the thyroid is evaluated. Once thyroid medication is started, a thyroid test should be completed at least every six months to monitor the medication dosing. These tests are for

- TSH: Thyroid-stimulating hormone—signaling hormone from the brain

- Free T4: Storage thyroid

- T3: Active thyroid

- Reverse T3: Competes for action at the cell site of T3 and can blunt the positive effects of active T3

- Thyroid antibodies:

  - TPO and TPG: antibodies for Hashimoto's disease

  - TSI and TR: antibodies for Graves' disease

There is a significant variance of opinion when interpreting what the thyroid's normal levels should be. However, here are some guidelines to keep in mind:

- TSH: Ideal level when taking thyroid medication is below 1.0–2.0

- Free T3 and free T4: Ideal level is mid to upper end of the normal range

- Reverse T3: Ideal level is mid to lower end of the normal range

- Do *not* take thyroid medications the day you are tested; fasting levels are best

- Consider adding supplements to optimize your levels if you need better results from a thyroid treatment.

Interpreting Thyroid Optimal Levels

This is the trickiest part of dealing with thyroid issues, primarily because of the wide range of opinions on how to treat or not treat thyroid disorders. If you were to line up 20 hormone, thyroid, and endocrine experts and asked them each their advice on how to treat hypothyroidism, you would probably get 20 different answers. So the key is to focus on the right treatment for you, which means working with a hormone specialist who will not only look at the labs but will also listen to you and work with you to get you to your optimal level, not just "normal."

The problem with diagnosing low thyroid is further complicated by the fact that opinions vary on the proper testing needed for low thyroid in the first place. The testing that is done most often in the US these days is a simple TSH (thyroid-stimulating hormone) test, which measures how the brain is signaling that it needs more thyroid hormone. This is often the only test that is ordered to evaluate the thyroid. (Talk about lazy medicine!) The problem with this is that TSH is only a signal coming from the brain—it can rise and fall daily or hourly. It is not the most conclusive way of testing for low thyroid or its possible underlying immune issues. Additionally, the TSH has a broad range (0.4–5.0 or higher), which means that if you have 10 out of 15 thyroid symptoms and this test comes back at 4.5 (remember, the higher number means your brain is calling for thyroid hormone to be made), you will likely be told you are perfectly normal when in fact your thyroid hormone levels are probably low. The full thyroid panel is worth asking for because it looks at the actual circulating levels in the blood so that the entire picture can be evaluated along with the symptoms.

One final issue with testing the thyroid specifically affects us brilliant women who are, shall we say, of a certain age. As women get older, low thyroid is often missed due to the loss of sensitivity of TSH in the blood. Research clearly shows that as you age, the TSH (signal from the brain) loses sensitivity, which means that a TSH level of 3.0 in an older woman (which most practitioners would call normal) corresponds to a much higher level in her younger years. Essentially, her numbers would reflect a normal thyroid while her symptoms got worse. The concerning issue with women as they age is that if they are not diagnosed, low thyroid will negatively affect memory and mood, and they will likely progress to a state where they are using many other drugs to treat their symptoms when all they need is thyroid hormone. Younger women under considerable stress are also a population often underdiagnosed, as many medical specialists are not thinking low thyroid could be a possibility in younger women. This is especially detrimental, as low thyroid in younger women leads to compromised growth and compromised development of the body and brain.

The big takeaway here is that thyroid disorders are greatly misunderstood in our culture. If you are suffering from a thyroid condition, you may have heard any of the following:

- You're lazy.

- Just eat less.

- Get out more.

- It's all in your head.

- Just get more sleep.

- Get it together!

The good news is that none of this is true, and there are steps you can take to feel better, which is exactly what we will explore throughout the remainder of this chapter.

FACTORS THAT AFFECT OPTIMAL THYROID FUNCTION

If the first part of this chapter left you feeling like walking into traffic, here's some good news: Simple nutrients can be used to greatly improve thyroid function, especially when it is low or borderline low. Some of these nutrients include: iron, iodine, selenium, and vitamins E, B2, B6, C, and D. Factors that can lower thyroid levels include stress, infections, medications, and toxins (like mercury, pesticides, and lead). With all this in mind, the main thing to consider when optimizing thyroid is the importance of converting storage thyroid T4 into active thyroid T3.

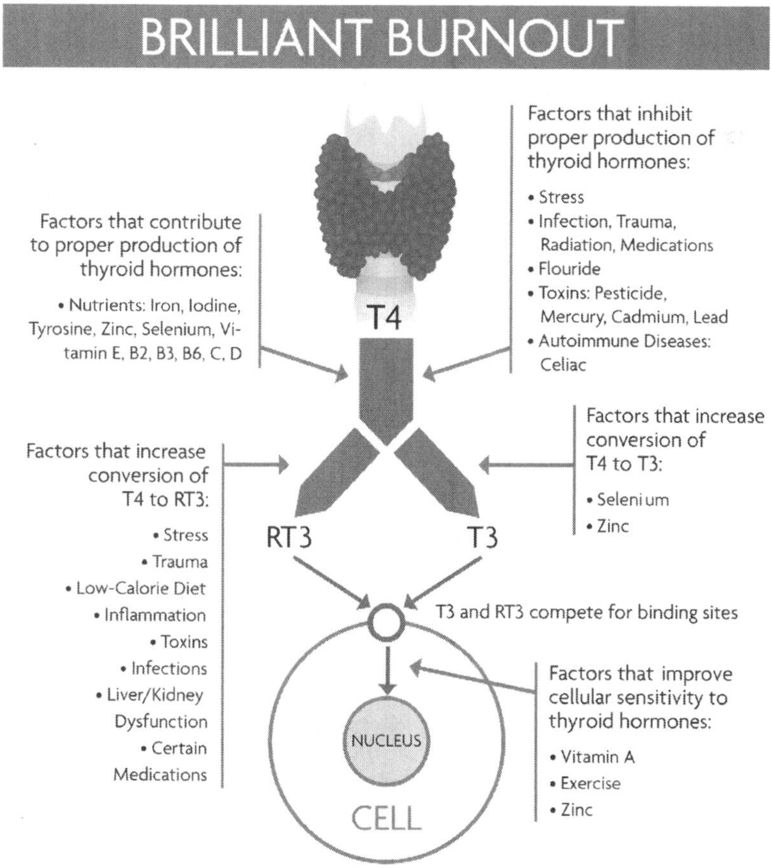

BRILLIANT BURNOUT

Factors that contribute to proper production of thyroid hormones:

• Nutrients: Iron, Iodine, Tyrosine, Zinc, Selenium, Vitamin E, B2, B3, B6, C, D

Factors that inhibit proper production of thyroid hormones:

• Stress
• Infection, Trauma, Radiation, Medications
• Flouride
• Toxins: Pesticide, Mercury, Cadmium, Lead
• Autoimmune Diseases: Celiac

T4

Factors that increase conversion of T4 to RT3:

• Stress
• Trauma
• Low-Calorie Diet
• Inflammation
• Toxins
• Infections
• Liver/Kidney Dysfunction
• Certain Medications

RT3   T3

Factors that increase conversion of T4 to T3:

• Selenium
• Zinc

T3 and RT3 compete for binding sites

Factors that improve cellular sensitivity to thyroid hormones:

• Vitamin A
• Exercise
• Zinc

NUCLEUS

CELL

Figure 4.1: Factors That Affect Thyroid Function

THYROID MEDICATION OPTIONS

There are many options for treating low thyroid with medication. The main types of thyroid medication options are

T4-only medications (these contain single T4 thyroid hormone only):

- Levothyroxine

- Synthroid

- Levoxyl

T3-only thyroid preparations (these contain T3 thyroid hormone only):

- Liothyronine

- Sustained release liothyronine (T3)

Desiccated thyroid medications containing T3 and T4 (animal derived):

- Armour thyroid

- WP thyroid

- Naturthroid

- NP thyroid

Factors Affecting Thyroid Medication

Many women (and men) taking thyroid medication have no idea that the other supplements or prescriptions they are taking could possibly interfere with the absorption of their thyroid medication. The following medications, supplements, and foods can interfere with the body's utilization of thyroid medication:

- Blood thinners, such as warfarin

- Estrogen-containing medications, such as birth control pills

- Sodium polystyrene sulfonate

- Antacids that contain aluminum hydroxide

- Calcium supplements

- Iron supplements and many multivitamins that contain iron

- Some cholesterol-lowering drugs

- Some foods may affect absorption as well, including soy products or very high fiber food

If you are regularly taking any of the above, consider talking to your health care provider about how you might optimize your thyroid balance or replace the other medication that could be interfering with absorption.

Natural vs. Synthetic Thyroid Medication— What's the Difference?

So, you got your thyroid tested, identified the problem, and are ready to start fixing it. But now you have to figure out which medication is best for you. It can seem like a daunting prospect, but stick with me. Here's what you need to know: Synthroid contains thyroxine, also called T4, and Cytomel contains T3, which is identical to the hormone produced by the thyroid gland. Levothyroxine is a generic form of Synthroid. It is produced by various other brand names worldwide, going by names such as Thyrax, Euthyrox, Levaxin, L-thyroxine, and Thyrox. Synthroid is bioidentical, but it's also synthetic. Natural thyroid pills are made from desiccated porcine (pig) thyroid glands that contain thyroxine (T4), T3, T2, T1, and calcitonin.

I know. Those were a lot of complicated words, but here's the big take-away: I personally feel no one combination is perfect for all hypothyroid or thyroid disorders. Clearly, using the best thyroid treatment for each person is imperative, and this treatment should be personalized not only to optimize the individual's levels but to relieve them of any symptoms. Sometimes this is easier achieved with a combination of Synthroid (T4) and Cytomel (T3), and at other times with desiccated thyroid, which contains the calcitonin that Synthroid does not contain.

I prefer to treat with T3 and T4 together, which means using either desiccated thyroid or the combination of Synthroid and Cytomel. Above all, I make sure that all my patients are converting T4 into T3 (which is often compromised with women under stress). I am against using Synthroid alone in the presence of low T3 levels (or elevated RT3 levels), especially if someone is symptomatic for low thyroid and/or has Hashimoto's thyroiditis.

Last, ensuring that the reverse T3 and the thyroid antibodies are in check as treatment ensues is vital. Working with each patient to support the entire thyroid-adrenal axis with lifestyle changes, supportive supplements, and diet can also not only help the patient feel better day to day, but it also supports the immune system.

Many specialists today claim a certain thyroid treatment is best, but all women are unique. What works for one may not work at all for the next, and medical providers should have many tools in their toolbox to fix imbalances on a case-by-case basis to achieve the best effects.

ADDITIONAL THYROID BALANCING OPTIONS

Sometimes it may happen that a patient follows all the right steps, identifying and treating their thyroid dysfunction with ruthless focus—but they still feel like crap. This is because sometimes a problem with the thyroid isn't *only* a problem with the thyroid. I like to teach each patient that in order to achieve balance, we must always be looking at our entire body, not just one gland or one problem area. All of our glands work together, and hormones must be in balance across the whole system in order to attain the best results. Some additional considerations for optimal thyroid balance are:

- Optimizing ferritin levels (adding iron when needed, which improves the conversion of T4 into active T3)

- Optimizing all hormone levels (especially progesterone, which is the supporting hormone to the thyroid)

- Optimizing pregnenolone (a hormone that is a precursor to all hormones)

- Checking for candida in the system to make sure there is *not* an overgrowth of yeast in the gut, preventing the right absorption of nutrients, minerals, and vitamins that support the thyroid (and of course the thyroid medication that they may be on), and adding a good probiotic to give the yeast some competition in the gut

- Making sure that reverse T3 is not elevated (robbing the benefits of the active T3 thyroid)

- Taking medication daily and preferably on an empty stomach separate from calcium, iron, and magnesium

- Knowing that all physicians and practitioners are not the same, and most today do not have the goal of "optimizing your thyroid"; they are mostly looking to see if the TSH is too high or too low

HASHIMOTO'S THYROIDITIS: THE NEW WAVE OF AUTOIMMUNE THYROID DISORDERS

The immune system is designed to attack and remove harmful invaders from the body, such as viruses, toxins, and bacteria. In women and men with an autoimmune disease, however, the immune system mistakes good cells for bad, and it attacks them by mistake. Hashimoto's thyroiditis happens when the immune system mistakenly sees normal thyroid gland cells as harmful and attacks them. Over time, your thyroid develops inflammation and often scarring and then fails to function. Hashimoto's thyroiditis is but one form of thyroiditis—an inflammation of the thyroid—that causes hypothyroidism, but it is also the most common type afflicting brilliant, highly stressed women.

Why this happens is unclear, but genetic factors, environmental factors, lifestyle habits, the immune system, and the health of the gut all appear to play a role. Hashimoto's disease can manifest in different ways, and early symptoms can be nonspecific and often are completely missed in the medical office, so patients with this condition are sometimes misdiagnosed or not diagnosed at all.

Conditions that may be confused with Hashimoto's include chronic fatigue, depression, anxiety, fibromyalgia, PMS, chronic pain, or insomnia. Unfortunately, when Hashimoto's is mistaken for one of these, it is then treated with medications that will not help the syndrome and, in many cases, will make it worse.

Triggers for Hashimoto's

Hashimoto's disease can be difficult to understand. There are triggers that can lead to the onset of this disease, and sufferers can become symptomatic over time. Some of these triggers include

- Genetic predispositions from gene mutation associated with HLA-DR3 or HLA-DR5

- Family history of thyroid disease

- Having another autoimmune disorder of any kind (often, people have several autoimmune disorders)

- Pregnancy and postpartum period (mostly due to stress and change of hormone levels)

- Excessive iodine intake (which is why iodine levels should be checked in the blood if someone is supplementing with iodine)

- Viral and bacterial infections or other illnesses that reduce, challenge, or overstress the immune system

- Epstein-Barr virus (the virus associated with mononucleosis)

- Hormone imbalances, deficiencies, or excess hormones

- Menopause, perimenopause, or significant imbalance in hormones during PMS

- Excessive ongoing stress that overtaxes the adrenals and compromises the HPA axis and the production of cortisol

- Excessive ongoing body inflammation due to poor diet, gluten intake, and lack of nutrients and antioxidants

- Lack of sleep (consistently less than seven hours per night of restorative sleep)

- Gut disorders, leaky gut, candida, small intestinal bacterial overgrowth (SIBO), and other disorders that compromise the immune system in the gut

The Connection between Excessive Stress and Autoimmune Disorders

In case you've become so engrossed in the intricacies of the thyroid that you've forgotten what this book is about, let me bring you back to the bigger issue here. A 2004 study in the journal *Thyroid* found that stress is one of the main environmental factors for thyroid autoimmunity.[13] Stressed-out adrenals can cause thyroid malfunction and possibly lead to an autoimmune crisis (the most prevalent rising autoimmune crisis we are facing today) when they become so overworked that they put the body in a state of catabolism, which means that the body is breaking down. When adrenals are overstressed, the body will slow down the thyroid gland as a protective mechanism. This may seem counterintuitive, but the reason behind this is that the thyroid gland controls the metabolism of the body, so the body has to slow it down in order to hold up the catabolic process. This is why, many times, the thyroid gland won't respond to treatment until you address any issues with the adrenal glands first. Ultimately, unaddressed issues in the adrenal glands can affect other bodily systems. For example, someone with weak adrenal glands who has a thyroid disorder can develop a compromised immune system, which can eventually lead to an autoimmune thyroid disorder, such as Hashimoto's hypothyroidism or thyroiditis. Also, when stressed, you're more vulnerable to autoimmune thyroid conditions (Hashimoto's thyroiditis) in general.

Symptoms of Hashimoto's Thyroiditis

Since the symptoms of Hashimoto's are similar to hypothyroidism, working with a specialist who can identify the differences between

---

13. Mark F. Prummel, Thea Strieder, and Wilmar M. Wiersinga, "The Environment and Autoimmune Thyroid Diseases," *European Journal of Endocrinology* 150 (2004): 605–618.

them is important. Some of the more specific symptoms of Hashimoto's are the following:

- Fatigue, often chronic and debilitating

- Weight gain or inability to lose weight

- Constipation, usually chronic and long term

- Sensitivity to cold, especially in the hands and feet

- Dry skin that usually worsens significantly in the winter months

- Depression and feelings of sadness or hopelessness

- Muscular aches, pains, and cramps that can sometimes be misdiagnosed as fibromyalgia or rheumatoid arthritis (or can exist alongside these two related autoimmune disorders)

- Reduced ability to tolerate exertion (e.g., fatigue on walking even short distances, inability to exercise, or feelings of lightheadedness when standing for too long)

- Irregular or extremely heavy menstrual periods

- Infertility or recurrent pregnancy loss

- Dry, brittle, and dull hair, skin, and nails

- Low basal body temperature

- Elevated LDL cholesterol

- Insomnia or fatigue, even after sleeping normal hours

- Anxiety, mood swings, and mood disorders (sometimes misdiagnosed as a major depressive disorder or bipolar disorder, but can exist alongside these conditions, too)

- Tenderness or pain in the lower throat where the thyroid sits, frequent sore throats not associated with sickness, or swelling of the throat, known as a goiter, or enlarged thyroid gland

- Increased susceptibility to viral or bacterial infections

- Increased incidence of diabetes

Testing for Hashimoto's

The only way to diagnose Hashimoto's is by a series of blood tests. Most doctors will run only a TSH test. You might recall, however, that TSH is not even a thyroid hormone but is produced by the pituitary gland in the brain to tell the thyroid to make more hormone. The assumption is that if your TSH is high, it means that your brain is shouting louder and louder at your thyroid to do its job, so there must be a problem with the thyroid.

This is where things get complicated. While that can certainly be true, other factors may be at play. The thyroid may not be producing the right levels of thyroid hormone because it is under attack from the immune system. The only way to deduce this condition is to test for thyroid antibodies—thyroid peroxidase antibody and thyroglobulin antibody. These antibodies play a primary role in the destruction of the thyroid by the immune system.

In order to get an accurate picture of what your thyroid is doing and whether you could have early, undiagnosed, or late-stage Hashimoto's, you need the following lab tests ordered:

- Free T3 (active form of T3)

- Free T4 (active form of T4)

- TSH

- Thyroglobulin antibodies

- Thyroid peroxidase antibodies

- Reverse T3 (a storage form of T3)

Treating Hashimoto's

Unfortunately, the battle for your health isn't over once you've received a proper diagnosis, not by a long shot. Many practitioners who even go so far as to correctly diagnose Hashimoto's thyroid disease will still stop short of a full-on treatment for the disorder. Instead, they will prescribe thyroid replacement and continue testing your thyroid levels until they normalize. But in many cases, while thyroid replacement can certainly take the edge off of symptoms or even totally neutralize them, it doesn't address the core issue as to why Hashimoto's started in the first place. Above all else, Hashimoto's is an immune problem, and until the immune system is calmed down, even if Hashimoto's enters remission, your body will be at risk for further autoimmune attacks.

A full-spectrum plan for Hashimoto's should involve further investigation as to what initially triggered the disorder as well as hormone replacement when needed. But it should also include dietary and lifestyle changes to remove any aggravating stressors that could be perpetuating the immune dysfunction and inflammation in the body. I like to use LDN (low-dose naltrexone) for Hashimoto's and most of the autoimmune syndromes that I encounter in the office. It is a safe compounded medication in a very low dose that has been shown to help release endorphins and reduce inflammation and antibody levels, as well as helping to reverse body pain, exhaustion, and depression. This is available through compounding pharmacies by prescription.

Hashimoto's Diet

Making dietary changes is your first line of defense in treating hypothyroidism and all hormone imbalances, especially those connected to stress. Many people with hypothyroidism experience crippling fatigue and brain fog, which typically prompts women to reach for non-nutritional forms of energy, like sugar and caffeine, comfort starch-like foods, and other quick fixes that only make them sicker. (Why, cake? Why would you betray me like this?)

A Hashimoto's diet should be one that first of all focuses on real, whole food. Processed food is filled with refined sugars and preservatives that will exacerbate inflammation and certainly not help restore balance to the immune system. Next, and of high importance, is the removal of gluten and dairy. As delicious as they may be, these two foods, when paired with leaky gut, can be enough to keep an autoimmune crisis running for years. When your gut is allowing undigested food particles into your bloodstream, the immune system misreads gluten in particular as thyroid tissue (because they're similar in structure), furthering the inflammation and autoimmune state. The immune system is insanely complex and intuitive in that it can produce cells to attack viruses, but it's not intelligent enough to understand what is self and what is non-self when it becomes compromised like this.

All this is to say that healing the gut lining is imperative to reach remission from Hashimoto's (or any autoimmune) disease. This means plenty of vegetables, good protein, high-quality omega-3 anti-inflammatory fats, and low-glycemic fruits. While all fruit certainly has its place, when you're under autoimmune attack, it's best to eat substantially more vegetables than fruits. Taking probiotics and obtaining adequate stool testing can also be of importance to ensure that the gut is healthy. Finally, keeping your blood sugar stable throughout the day and not overeating is critical to reducing the work the body is having to do to digest. Always remember that the body will heal best when it is balanced.

NUTRIENTS THAT SUPPORT OUR THYROID

The thyroid gland needs specific vitamins and minerals to properly do its job. This seems like an easy fix—just swallow a handful of multivitamins, right? It's not quite that simple. Because how our hormones function is unique to each of us, the best way to get a handle on what our body specifically needs is to have a full thyroid panel done to help pinpoint where individual levels may be off balance. Research shows us that a few key nutrients are highly valuable for everyone.

Iodine

This is the most important trace element vital to thyroid functioning. Without iodine, the thyroid does not have the basic building blocks it needs to make the necessary hormones to support all of the tissues in the body. Iodine-rich foods include sea vegetables, kelp, seafood (such as haddock, clams, salmon, shrimp, oysters, and sardines) iodized sea salt, eggs, spinach, garlic, asparagus, Swiss chard, mushrooms, summer squash, sesame seeds, and lima beans.

Selenium

This mineral is indispensable to our thyroid in several ways. Selenium-containing enzymes protect the thyroid gland when we are under stress, working like a detox to help flush oxidative, chemical, and even social stress, which can cause adverse reactions in our body. Selenium-based proteins also help regulate hormone synthesis, converting T4 into the more accessible T3. Some foods that are loaded with selenium are tuna, mushrooms, beef, sunflower seeds, brazil nuts, organ meats, halibut, and soybeans.

Vitamin A

This vitamin is also needed for thyroid manufacturing and can be found in foods such as broccoli, asparagus, lettuce, kale, carrots, spinach, sweet potatoes, liver, winter squash or pumpkin, and cantaloupe.

Copper

This mineral is needed to help produce TSH and to maintain T4 production. T4 helps cholesterol regulation, and some research even indicates copper deficiency may contribute to higher cholesterol and heart issues for people with hypothyroidism. Don't go sucking on doorknobs to get this, though. Instead, eat foods rich in this mineral, such as crabmeat, oysters, lobster, beef, nuts, sunflower seeds, beans (white beans, chickpeas, soybeans), shiitake mushrooms, pearled barley, tomato paste, and dark chocolate.

Iron

Decreased levels of iron can result in decreased thyroid function as well. When combined with an iodine deficiency, iron must be replaced to repair the thyroid imbalance. Iron-rich foods include organ meats, oysters, clams, spinach, lentils, soybeans, white beans, pumpkin seeds, and blackstrap molasses.

Zinc

Low levels of zinc can cause T4, T3, and the thyroid-stimulating hormone (TSH) to also become low. Zinc-rich foods include: beef, turkey, lamb, fresh oysters, sardines, soybeans, walnuts, sunflower seeds, Brazil nuts, pecans, almonds, split peas, ginger root, and maple syrup.

FAST TRACK: REBOOTING YOUR THYROID FUNCTION

Now that you have a more in-depth overview of the thyroid and how it affects every area of the body, we can simply put together a fast-track plan to plug any hole present that could be causing you to drag yourself around with an empty tank.

- Seek out a hormone-balancing expert and ask for a full thyroid panel. This includes all of the tests listed in this chapter, and be conscientious to ensure that you are in the mid to upper end of normal range for T3 and T4 and not right on the brink of abnormally low. (See Appendix G for suggestions on finding a hormone expert.)

- Repeat testing every three months until optimal levels have been achieved and every six months thereafter, ensuring all hormones from the ovaries, adrenals, and thyroid are balanced and optimal. (Remember, all of these systems work together.)

- STOP the sugar, starch, and flour. This is a vital step. Start reading labels, and try to reduce these inflammatory foods in your diet that keep you feeling awful.

- Eat veggies to your heart's content and keep stocked up on them.

- Increase lean, organic proteins in the diet. Protein transports thyroid hormone to all your tissues and stabilizes your blood sugar levels, helping to calm the entire stress system. Proteins include nuts and nut butters, quinoa, hormone- and antibiotic-free animal products (organic, grass-fed meats, eggs, and sustainably farmed fish), and legumes.

- If you are a vegan, be *very* careful that you are not making your health worse by only eating carbs and soy. This could be making you even more sick. Isoflavones in soybeans can inhibit the enzyme that adds iodine to the thyroid hormone known as thyroid perox-idase (TPO). Studies indicate that excessive soy isoflavone might bond with the iodine we do have, diminishing the reserve for thy-roid production. The issue lies with the levels of iodine we have. If levels are sufficient, eating natural soy should not be a problem.

- Increase the intake of healthy fats. That's right—fat is your friend. Fats are essential for hormone production, as hormones are made from fat. Natural, healthy fats include olive oil, avocados, flax seeds, fish, nuts, nut butters, hormone- and antibiotic-free full-fat cheese, yogurt, cottage cheese, and coconut milk products.

- Add essential vitamins and nutrients to your diet, especially vitamin D (ask for vitamin D testing and make sure your level is between 50–80 ng/ml), B complex, high-dose vitamin C, omega-3 fatty acids, selenium, zinc, copper, and vitamin A.

- Stay away from dairy. Lactose can be an issue for many women, as they often do not tolerate lactose as they age or if they have any immune compromise at the gut level. Some specialists feel that hypothyroidism is closely connected to several gut disorders, including celiac disease. Lactose (dairy) intake in some cases can even elevate TSH levels, creating an imbalance and suboptimal thy-roid hormone production.

- Eliminate gluten. The chemical composition of gluten is nearly the same as thyroid tissue, and with inflammatory autoimmune disor-ders like Hashimoto's, eating gluten is like putting fuel to the fire, as the body will attack the thyroid even more, creating havoc and more symptoms of fatigue and pain. This will keep you in an auto-immune state, which is not good for anyone.

- Use herbs, such as sage, ashwagandha, waterhyssop, and forskolin combined with iodine and selenium. These herbs can help boost energy and support a healthy metabolism.

- Start changing your lifestyle to get into an anti-inflammatory, healthy state.

  - Get at least 8–9 hours of restful sleep per night.

  - Make yourself stop when you have reached your limit of stress for the day; then, take a walk and clear your head (even if it is only for ten minutes).

  - Breathe deeply and regularly. Stop holding your breath; this will cause stress alarms to go off.

  - Hydrate yourself. Often.

  - Consider fasting at least 13 hours per day, starting after dinner and going into the next day. Do not eat late at night. Every time you eat, you are asking your body to exert more energy to digest. Instead, give your gastrointestinal system a break from early in the evening till the next day so your body can focus on regenerating and rebooting its hormones and brain chemicals while you sleep.

When we support our thyroid naturally, we can improve the way we feel on many levels. It may seem complicated, but once we learn which foods help and how to support our thyroid with the micronutrients we need, it will become second nature.

Thyroid Reboot Success Story

Jackie D. was the kind of woman we all admire (and maybe secretly envy). She was a long-distance runner, she loved to stay busy, and she always volunteered for everything. She was so good at it that she became the one gal everyone could depend on to get the job done, so Jackie piled on the stress every day. She loved running and often competed in triathlons and marathons. Being so athletic, she never struggled with her weight or energy, but right after turning 36 she noticed that her belly was getting fat, she had lost her ability to get past midafternoon without hitting a wall, and she didn't feel like her spunky self any longer.

She was having a difficult time concentrating and managing projects and began to feel unmotivated and depressed. Her periods became erratic and heavy, and she would often spend one week a month just recovering from her heavy period the week before. She forced herself to keep running, but this was suddenly taking a toll. She had increasing levels of body pain, weakness, and a complete loss of endurance. She was a vegan and mostly ate carbohydrates, with her only source of protein being soy. As she began to feel worse, she started eating more comfort (sugary) foods and snacking on crackers, chips, and other foods that she normally never ate. She finally went to her OB/GYN who tested her TSH and found it was 4.5. This, her doctor told her, was perfectly normal. But she knew she was not normal. She was starting to feel desperate and, by the time she showed up at my office, was lamenting the fact that she just wanted her life back the way it used to be.

We ran a full panel on Jackie, and since her visit to the OB/GYN, her TSH had risen to 6.0 with low T3 at 2.3 and suboptimal T4 at 0.6. Even more telling was that she had elevated antibodies (autoimmune Hashimoto's), which explained why she felt so poor. We talked at length about how to get her balanced, utilizing a full-body approach, and she was more than willing to do whatever it took. She was ready to get her fight back.

Her game plan included the following:

- Immediately starting on thyroid medication to keep those hormones in the optimal ranges

- Eating a balanced diet focusing on

  - Incorporating more protein sources

  - Eliminating soy

  - Increasing nutrients to support the entire endocrine system

- Being mindful of the stress in her life due to its effects on her thyroid

- Optimizing her low testosterone level

- Optimizing her low progesterone level

- Starting on a low-dose naltrexone (compounded LDN) to provide ammunition against the autoimmune cycle

In only 90 days, she was nearly back to normal. She had sustained energy throughout the day, no body pain, regular menstrual cycles, no depression, and better concentration and memory. She was even back to running again, but she decided to take it easy and not push herself as hard by adding yoga, strength training, and stretching into her routine. She was so inspired by her recovery, in fact, that she became an advocate for other women suffering from stress-induced hypothyroidism and Hashimoto's. She is forever grateful for her second chance at life. Above all, she now understands how to keep it all in check to feel her best.

5

Brilliant Brain Balance: Losing Your Mind and Mood with Stress and How to Break Through

"I put my heart and my soul into my work and have lost my mind in the process."
—VAN GOGH

In this chapter, we're going to explore the role stress plays on your mood. Take the quiz that follows to see if your brain is balanced.

QUIZ: IS YOUR BRAIN OFF BALANCE?

1. Do you have a tendency to be pessimistic and negative, to see the glass as half empty rather than half full? Y/N

2. Are you often worried and anxious? Y/N

3. Are you often obsessive? Is it hard for you to be flexible? Are you a perfectionist or a control freak? Y/N

4. Are you apt to be irritable, impatient, edgy, or angry? Y/N

5. Have you had anxiety or panic attacks? Y/N

6. Do you get PMS or menopausal moodiness (tears, anger, depression)? Y/N

7. Have you had fibromyalgia (unexplained muscle pain) or TMJ (pain, tension, and grinding associated with your jaw)? Y/N

8. Do you often feel depressed—the flat, bored, apathetic kind of depression? Y/N

9. Do you have difficulty focusing or concentrating or have you been diagnosed with ADD? Y/N

10. Do you often feel overworked, pressured, or constantly under a deadline? Y/N

11. Do you have trouble relaxing or loosening up? Y/N

12. Does your body tend to be stiff, uptight, tense? Y/N

13. Are you easily upset, frustrated, or snappy under stress? Y/N

14. Do you often feel overwhelmed or as though you just can't get it all done? Y/N

15. Do you feel weak or shaky at times? Y/N

16. Do you use tobacco, alcohol, food, or drugs to relax and calm down? Y/N

17. Do you tend to avoid dealing with painful issues? Y/N

18. Do you use drugs such as methadone, OxyContin, codeine, or other opiates? Y/N

19. Have you been through a great deal of physical or emotional pain? Y/N

20. Do you suffer from chronic back pain or headaches? Y/N

21. Do you crave pleasure, comfort, reward, enjoyment, or numbing from treats like chocolate, bread, wine, romance novels, marijuana, tobacco, or lattes? Y/N

If you answered yes to at least three of these questions, you may need a brain chemical balancing plan to support your neurochemicals. This is nothing to be ashamed of. You're not crazy; you're just human. And when we humans try to deal with too much stress, it isn't hard to lose our minds. But now I'm going to teach you how to get your brain back.

WHAT ARE NEUROCHEMICALS?

Our brains are so complex that it's simply not possible to even conceive of their intricacies. (And yes, I hear the irony in that, but it's true.) It's hard to describe the complexity of the truly awesome network of cells that make up your nervous system and brain. But I'm going to try anyway. The average brain houses over 100 billion cells, each connected to thousands of other cells that create trillions of connections in your brain. This means that everything we do, think, or create is a result of these nerve cells communicating with each other via electrical, chemical, and hormonal pathways. The nerve cells (neurons) talk to each other across these connections though specialized chemicals called neurotransmitters. These messengers are mostly made in the gastrointestinal tract but exert their effect on the brain and work to coordinate the discussions needed between cells to achieve the right thought, action, or movement in the body. The brain chemicals interact with target sites located throughout the body and brain to help regulate emotions like fear, pleasure, anger, and joy and also help with mood, memory, concentration, energy, appetite, pain control, cravings, and sleep. These amazing tiny messengers are chemicals that link the brain and spinal cord to the body (muscles, organs, and glands) and affect every cell, tissue, and system in the body. Because this is such a complex set of interactions that also integrate with the entire endocrine system (including the adrenals), many things can go wrong if it is off balance—or if you are overstressed.

Some of the problems that can occur if the neurotransmitters are off balance or depleted are the following

- Anxiety

- Insomnia

- Fatigue

- Pain

- Obesity

- Mood disorders

- Addictions

- Hormone disruptions

THE BALANCING ACT

Proteins, minerals, vitamins, fats, and carbohydrates are all essential nutrients that your brain needs to manufacture adequate levels of the neurotransmitters that regulate your mood and overall emotional and mental balance. These neurotransmitters are mostly made in the gastrointestinal (gut) tract, but the bulk of their effects are on the brain. A disruption anywhere in this process due to poor diet, excessive stress, or a lack of good self-care can quickly lead to mood disruptions like depression, irritability, and anxiety. The four major neurotransmitters that regulate mood are serotonin, dopamine, GABA, and norepinephrine. In addition to this, there are two main types of neurotransmitters: inhibitory and excitatory. These all work together to build a web of complex interactions full of checks and balances in an attempt to keep the system in line at all times.

Inhibitory (Calming) Neurotransmitters

The following "cool down" your nervous system:

GABA

Gamma-aminobutyric acid is your calming neurotransmitter. It is considered the "natural Xanax" of the brain. Because of this, the GABA neurotransmitter system is where most sedatives, prescription sleep aids, and tranquilizers work. GABA helps the neurons recover after firing to keep anxiety and worry at bay. When under stress, GABA works to keep things cool, calm, and downregulated.

Anxiety sets in when this system is not well supported and signals are lost, muted, or misfired. Excessive, ongoing stress can often cause this, which results in anxiety overrides. If GABA is overproduced (which can happen with high stress), you will feel sluggish and sleepy with brain fog (as if you were recovering from a high-adrenaline stressful incident). If GABA is deficient in the system, it can lead to anxiety, impulsivity, restlessness, irritability, and an overall inability to handle stress.

SEROTONIN

Serotonin is referred to as the master neurotransmitter. It controls our mood, sleep, digestion, appetite, sexual desire, concentration, pain perception, and learning ability. (Talk about multipurpose!) High levels of stress, lack of sleep, poor nutrition, inflammation, genetic mutations, and prescription medications can all cause an imbalance in serotonin and slowly reduce its levels, leading to poor mood, depression, worry, insomnia, compulsive behavior, sugar or carb cravings, obsessive thoughts, PMS, headaches, irritable bowels, and body pain. Low serotonin levels will also interfere with the conversion of T4 thyroid into active T3 thyroid hormone, furthering any fatigue and depression. Serotonin is critical to feelings of self-worth and happiness and helps protect against depression and anxiety.

Excitatory (Stimulating) Neurotransmitters

The following stimulate and "fire up" the nervous system:

DOPAMINE

Dopamine functions as both an inhibitory and excitatory transmitter. Adequate dopamine levels are needed to allow you to focus and concentrate on a given task. As such, attention deficit problems stem from low or faulty dopamine levels. Dopamine is also the main player in regulating the reward and pleasure centers of the brain. (This is why it plays such a huge role with addictions.) This neurotransmitter is also critical for memory and motor skills.

Low dopamine levels (which reduce the sense of well-being) are quite common and often go years without diagnosis or treatment. Dopamine is responsible for sheer motivation, interest, and the drive to achieve. When levels are low, you lose your zest and enthusiasm for life, experience great difficulty completing tasks, and have poor concentration and no energy. Low levels of dopamine are often seen with any type of drug addiction because the drugs burn out your body's supply. Drugs prescribed for attention deficit disorder (ADD) or attention deficit hyperactivity disorder (ADHD) will temporarily address symptoms of low dopamine by pushing your existing supply into the space between two neurons (the synapse). This will often work in the short run, but using these prescription drugs for any length of time could (and often does) inhibit the natural transmission and production of dopamine.

EPINEPHRINE

Epinephrine, also known as adrenaline, is a neurotransmitter and hormone that is essential to metabolism. It regulates attention, mental focus, arousal, and brain function. It is made from norepinephrine and is released by the adrenal glands. If your body produces an excessive amount of epinephrine, you will find yourself feeling anxious and hyperactive, you will be unable to get to sleep or stay asleep, and you will have an overall miserable feeling. If you have low levels of epinephrine, then you will feel run down, apathetic, foggy, unmotivated, fatigued, and flat.

PEA

Phenethylamine (PEA) is a transmitter made from phenylalanine. It is important in focus and concentration. High levels of this can cause a racing mind, insomnia, anxiety, and a revved-up feeling. Low PEA can cause difficulty with attention span, low moods, depression, apathy, and a reduced ability to focus.

NOREPINEPHRINE

This is the counterpart to epinephrine (adrenaline), and its primary purpose is arousal. When you are stressed, norepinephrine will cause you to be more aware, awake, and attentive. It helps you focus on the task at hand. Depression can be caused from many factors related to neurotransmitter imbalance, with the most common being low serotonin, but it can also be caused by low norepinephrine, which would explain why antidepressants only work in half of the population who take them (since antidepressants often work on serotonin levels only). With low levels of norepinephrine, one might feel depressed and lacking focus and attention. High levels are often associated with mania, overexcitement, hyperfocus, or the inability to settle down.

WHY BRILLIANT WOMEN NEED OPTIMAL BRAIN CHEMICAL BALANCE

So, here's the bottom line: Without our brains, we wouldn't be brilliant. Pretty obvious, right? We have to keep our brains working at the best possible level or our ability to overachieve and stay in the game is simply not going to happen. This is the crux of who we are, and I want to help you keep it that way. I want to enlighten you on what it takes to turn your current stressed, off-balance brain into one that is fully functional for years to come, keeping you performing at the highest level with the least amount of emotional and mental breakdowns.

First, let's talk about what excessive stress does to the brain.

8 WAYS STRESS AFFECTS YOUR BRAIN

1. Stress depletes you of precious brain chemicals like serotonin and dopamine, causing depression and anxiety. Serotonin is the happy brain chemical that also plays a role in mood, learning, appetite, and sleep. Low serotonin is directly related to depression and anxiety, and low dopamine causes a lack of zest, enthusiasm, and motivation for life and is the primary factor in addictions.

2. Stress halts the production of new brain cells, which explains why when we are overly stressed we don't always think clearly or act in our best interests. Brain-derived neurotrophic factor (BDNF) is a protein that's essential for keeping brain cells healthy, but high-stress cortisol production or stress hormone imbalances reduce the production of BDNF, resulting in a halted production of new brain cells. The good news is that putting a stop to this imbalance means that, as you age, you can still make new, healthy brain cells. (Thank goodness!)

3. Chronic stress creates brain fog and emotional instability. Memory problems and a lack of concentration and focus are the hallmarks of chronic stress. Research clearly shows that chronic high stress causes electrical signals in the brain to be delayed or compromised, leaving us wondering why we walked into the bathroom only seconds after we knew we had to go pee.

4. Stress increases the radical damage in our brain. With high stress, free radicals (killer molecules) are made in surplus, which can cause normal healthy brain cells to rupture and die. If this is coupled with lack of sleep, poor diet, and excessive nutrient deficiencies, the free radical formation increases even more.

5. Stress makes your brain small. Yes, you heard that right. Research continues to show that high stress halts the making of new brain cells and neuronal pathways in the brain. Stress literally shrinks areas like the hippocampus (an area important for memory and emotions) and the prefrontal cortex (an area important for decision making and impulsive behavior).

6. Stress increases the chances you will have Alzheimer's and dementia. One in three US seniors will die with Alzheimer's or some form of dementia. So we should be careful to protect our brains.

7. Stress can lead to a toxic waste site in the brain. Every cell in our body is sensitive to toxins, but the brain is on the top of the list when it comes to sensitivity. We have a brain filter that normally keeps us safe, but when this barrier is compromised with stress, causing it to be "leaky," it lets in pathogens, poisons like heavy metals, chemicals, and other toxins we are exposed to.

8. Stress causes the brain to become inflamed. There are special cells in the brain called microglia that protect the brain from infection and toxins. Essentially, they are part of the brain's immune system. Unfortunately, with high, relentless stress, these microglia overreact, causing inflammation. This inflammation seems to have a role in all areas of disease in the body and can lead to depression.

HOW BRAIN CHEMICALS ARE AFFECTED BY STRESS

The thing that really blows my mind (pun intended) is that millions of women are suffering silently from anxiety, low-lying depression, brain scramble, cravings, and loss of memory to the point that they think they really do have dementia or Alzheimer's. Apparently, we have an epidemic on our hands with a skyrocketing number of people suffering from these disorders, but women in particular are hardly ever offered a thorough evaluation of their brain chemicals or even a discussion on what might be happening with them. Instead, they are usually prescribed an antidepressant. These women are told, "See you in a few months" and are referred to counseling. Really? That's the best we can do?

When it comes to the brain, most psychiatrists and general practitioners focus on depression and medications to fix the ailments or symptoms of it but rarely look at the entire person to figure out what needs to be done to fix the underlying issues. Where they should be looking is at the neurotransmitters. Neurotransmitters are vitally important in the stress response because they allow us to cope with everyday stressors with a clear mind, they promote good mental performance, and they grant us the needed motor skills to move through our day with a balanced emotional outlook.

Everyone suffers from intermittent blues or feeling down, but increased, ongoing high stress can compromise the integrity of the brain's neurotransmitter balance. This leaves you with a serious deteriorated emotional and mental state that can create day-to-day concerns and an inability to cope. Anxiety and depression often occur when you know that the demands from your environment are greater than your capacity to deal with them. High, daily occurring stress causes you to feel worse emotionally. Mentally, you are not reacting as you normally would, and your neurotransmitters are likely off balance. Unfortunately, if this imbalance is not dealt with, it can destroy your entire sense of well-being over time.

The Cortisol-Dopamine-Serotonin Connection

Research continues to show that stress-induced depression and anxiety are on the rise. Of those individuals who are clinically depressed, about one half will have an excess of cortisol in their blood early on, with subsequent very low levels of cortisol, leaving them with depression and an inability to manage stress. When the endocrine system is functioning properly, the hypothalamus monitors the amount of cortisol that is released by the adrenal gland. When cortisol levels rise, the hypothalamus slows down its influence on the pituitary gland by decreasing the production of hormones it releases. Conversely, when cortisol levels drop, the hypothalamus stimulates ACTH production and the release of cortisol. However, in depressed individuals, the hypothalamus may continuously influence the pituitary gland to produce ACTH without regard for cortisol levels. (Can you say imbalance?)

Other research concerning cortisol has shown that the timing of the release of this hormone may be problematic in those who are depressed.[14] People who are not depressed tend to secrete cortisol at certain times of the day. Normally, cortisol levels are highest at approximately 8:00 a.m. and lowest at night. This normal cycling of cortisol levels does not occur in some people who are depressed. For instance, they might have consistent, low levels of cortisol throughout the day and high levels in the middle of the night, compromising their sleep and recovery.

With prolonged stress, cortisol decreases the amino acid tryptophan, which is necessary for serotonin production. This is especially bad because, as you now know, serotonin prevents depression and helps you feel happy. It also has an effect on appetite, sleep, and sexual desire, so not having enough of it can be a real downer.

Most antidepressants block the destruction and re-uptake of serotonin, which temporarily increases serotonin levels. But, eventually, the

---

14 "All About Depression," October 19, 2018, http://www.allaboutdepression.com/index.html.

adrenal glands slow down (out of survival) and the production of cortisol declines, which leads to worsening depression. When cortisol declines, the ability to mobilize glucose for energy also decreases. This decline leads to fatigue, impaired brain function, and further imbalance of neurotransmitters. The lack of cortisol also activates the SNS, which leads to more anxiety and an inability to handle stress.

Patients with Cushing's syndrome, whose adrenal glands produce excessive cortisol, often have depression and anxiety. In addition, patients who are on high doses of cortisol to treat conditions such as lupus and rheumatoid arthritis can develop depression after prolonged therapy. Repeated or chronic exposure to stress, rather than short-term stress, puts an individual at a huge risk of developing depression and anxiety.

The Downward Spiral of Using Prescription Medications for Brain Imbalance

We now know that common medications and our everyday habits cause the body imbalance in many ways. We are seeing more and more side effects from loss of vitamins, minerals, and nutrient levels caused by medications that block them. We are also seeing the side effects of prescription drugs on the gut. These drugs can block the effects of other supplements or hormones or even directly and negatively impact the immune system. We also know that medications that affect the brain might also affect other areas of the body. The bottom line here is that if you are experiencing intense demands on your life and have noticed that your stress is causing you to feel anxious, depressed, unmotivated, down, or lacking attention, focus, and alertness, then you likely need a full stress hormone reboot and not a prescription medication that could possibly cause more serious long-term side effects. It's at least worth considering. All this being said, I would like to dig in a little deeper on the two common categories of drugs prescribed to women who are exceedingly stressed, which can exacerbate a brain chemical imbalance.

ANTIDEPRESSANTS

Antidepressant medications are the most commonly prescribed treatment for depression and are now often used to treat post-traumatic stress disorder (PTSD), OCD, pain syndromes, menopause, autoimmune syndromes, substance abuse, PMS, anxiety, and eating disorders. Most antidepressants are designed to alter levels of serotonin or dopamine or both. In the brain, serotonin acts as a chemical that controls the firing of neurons that help us think, feel, and behave, and in this way antidepressants can be helpful. However, serotonin regulates many other processes in other parts of the body, including digestion, muscle control, blood clotting, and reproductive health.

Most antidepressants are intended to bind to molecules in the brain called *transporters* that regulate neurotransmitters like serotonin. When they bind to transporters, they help prevent the reabsorption of serotonin, which then causes a buildup of serotonin outside the neurons, thereby easing the feelings of depression. Unfortunately, when antidepressants travel throughout the body, they bind to a serotonin transporter wherever it is found, which inevitably interferes with processes in other parts of the body where serotonin is found.

Because medical doctors and practitioners are focused on the mood effects of antidepressants, often the other potential problems are not brought up and discussed (like digestion, sexual functioning, abnormal fertility, and menstrual bleeding issues). Another problem is that as the serotonin increases outside the cell, the brain begins to resist the effects of the antidepressants over time, which can lead to needing higher dosages or a stronger combination of drugs in order to get a better effect.

Antidepressants have also been shown to alter testosterone levels in the blood, causing problems with sex drive and function in men and women.[15] Studies also show that antidepressants cause significant cognitive decline over time, impair driving performance and increase car accidents, and can

---

15 Alan J. Cohen, "Antidepressant-Induced Sexual Dysfunction Associated with Low Serum Free Testosterone," *Mental Health Today* (2000), http://www.mental-health-today.com/rx/testos.htm.

significantly reduce memory and cognitive thinking in older individuals.[16] Antidepressants are also associated with impaired gastrointestinal functioning, as they increase the serotonin in the intestinal lining (you have many serotonin receptors in the gut), which can lead to irritable bowel syndrome, pain, diarrhea, constipation, indigestion, and bloating.

All this is to say that women need a thorough evaluation of their mood and brain symptoms to identify the best course of treatment and not to simply accept a potentially harmful medication because it's convenient. When we are depressed, anxious, or we can't sleep, a personalized approach for treatment is of utmost importance. We should carefully and thoroughly examine the entire system to figure out what is off balance and could lead to these problems. Resorting to the use of a drug that may create even more issues is not the answer. Sometimes these medications can help, but we should always dig a little deeper first.

ATTENTION DEFICIT DRUGS

Another growing class of drugs that many adults (including a frighteningly large number of young women) are using to mentally stay in the game are the drugs used to treat ADD. The problem is that nearly anyone can get these drugs. They are widely prescribed if your attention and memory are not what they used to be, and it is quite easy to intentionally test positive for ADD to get a prescription. (To be clear, I'm not advocating that. Lying to a doctor is pretty much always a bad idea.) ADD drugs increase your energy, reduce your appetite, increase your motivation, and help you achieve laser focus so you can get more done on your to-do list. Sounds kind of like they bottled what makes us brilliant. What's not to like about all of that?

A lot, it turns out. Recent research shows that these medications may damage the nucleus accumbens, an area of the brain that is crucial to

---

16 Mehdi Sayyah, Kaveh Eslami, Shabnam AlaiShehni, and Leila Kouti, "Cognitive Function before and during Treatment with Selective Serotonin Reuptake Inhibitors in Patients with Depression or Obsessive-Compulsive Disorder," *Psychiatry Journal* (2016), doi: 10.1155/2016/5480391.

motivation and drive.[17] What happens to the serotonin transporters with antidepressants can also happen with dopamine transporters on ADD drugs. If you develop more dopamine transporters (due to taking medications that potentiate this), then ultimately the dopamine will be "taken up more freely" by the body, leaving you with the need for more. This is why it is very difficult to stop taking these medications once you start. And you often need a higher dose over time to achieve the same effect. This is particularly a problem if a person suddenly stops taking the medication or tries to lower the dose. The dopamine is still getting cleared more quickly, leaving you feeling unmotivated, unfocused, and uninterested and unable to get through the day. This can lead to severe inattention and the need for higher, more potent dosing.

These days, people experience a lack of attention, focus, or mental stamina for so many reasons. And while ADD is a real syndrome, don't you think it would be wiser to balance the brain chemicals that actually need it with amino acids, or to optimize the hormones to activate the brain, or to recalibrate the stress hormone cortisol to fix the problem? I do!

THE EFFECTS OF ALCOHOL ON THE BRAIN

We hear many different things about how alcohol affects the brain and body, most notably that it is a depressant, but that's only part of the story. It is a depressant, but weirdly enough it's also an indirect stimulant. It also plays a few other roles that might surprise you. Alcohol directly affects brain chemistry by altering levels of neurotransmitters—the chemical messengers that transmit the signals throughout the body that control thought processes, behavior, and emotion. Alcohol affects both excitatory and inhibitory neurotransmitters.

---

17 Steven M. Berman, Ronald Kuczenski, and Edythe D. London, "Potential Adverse Effects of Amphetamine Treatment on Brain and Behavior: a Review," *Molecular Psychiatry* 15 (2010): 1121–1122, doi: 10.1038/mp2010.39.

An example of an excitatory neurotransmitter is glutamate, which would normally increase brain activity and energy levels. Alcohol suppresses the release of glutamate, resulting in a slowdown along your brain's highways. An example of an inhibitory neurotransmitter is GABA, which reduces energy levels and calms everything down. Drugs like Xanax and Valium (and other benzodiazepines) increase GABA production in the brain, resulting in sedation. Alcohol also has a unique effect on GABA, and it's one that ties in directly to the unhealthy ways we often deal with stress.

The Alcohol-Stress Connection

With stress comes some level of anxiety, which, as many of us know all too well, alcohol easily manages. Alcohol increases the effects of GABA in the brain, creating a sense of calmness. What this means for you is that your thoughts, speech, and movements are slowed down, and the more you drink, the more of these effects you'll feel (hence the stumbling around, falling over chairs, and other clumsy things drunk people do). But here's the twist: Alcohol also increases the release of dopamine in your brain's reward center. The reward center is the same combination of brain areas (the ventral striatum) that are affected by virtually all pleasurable activity, including everything from hanging out with friends to getting a big bonus at work or even having sex. By jacking up dopamine levels in your brain, alcohol tricks you into thinking that it's making you feel great (or maybe just better if you are drinking to get over something emotionally difficult). The effect is that you keep drinking to get your brain to release more dopamine, but at the same time you're altering other brain chemicals that are enhancing your feelings of depression.

Over time, with more drinking, the dopamine effect diminishes until it's almost nonexistent. But at this stage, a drinker is often hooked on the feeling of dopamine release in the reward center, even though they're no longer getting it. Once a compulsive need to go back again and again for that release is established, addiction takes hold. The length of time it takes for this to happen is case specific. Some people have a genetic propensity for alcoholism, and for them it will take very little time, while for others it may take several weeks, months, or even years.

Moderation

I understand the joys of social drinking and how difficult it can be not to have a drink to wind down. But we have to keep our brain in balance, and moderation will help with this. It also helps make sure you are constantly balanced with other neurotransmitters in the brain, gut, and body. Even taking an amino acid supplement to support serotonin if you do drink socially will help with the balance of serotonin and dopamine and help keep you more in control.

Again, our focus should be on protecting our brain, because without this precious, valuable, and irreplaceable organ, we would be totally screwed. Keeping our brain chemicals in check and the neurotransmitters balanced is the goal for optimal concentration, memory, mood, and focus. Habituating on anything that alters the brain in a negative way is the fast pass to long-term problems that often are not reversible.

THE NOT-SO-BRILLIANT BURNOUT DIET

The brain only weighs about three pounds, but it takes a whopping 20 percent of your total daily calorie intake to run it. This is why a brain-healthy diet is essential for keeping your memory and intellect sharp and your mood lifted. We often joke about how women eat their feelings, but now we know this might actually be a backward statement. A new study published in the *American Journal of Clinical Nutrition* found that eating foods high in sugar and starch is likely to increase a person's risk for depression.[18] The same goes for eating high amounts of added sugars as well as refined grains, so next time you're tempted to go to the donut store, remember: It will only make you sadder. The good news is that the same study found that foods high in fiber, like fruits and vegetables, are associated with a significantly lower risk of depression.

Another large, rather disturbing study called the Women's Health Initiative (WHI) observational study came out in 2001 and examined the lifestyle and hormone habits of 93,000 women, ages 50–79. This study rocked the world of women taking hormones, and in my opinion wrongly convinced many women to stop taking all their hormones, instead of only the problem hormone revealed in the study (synthetic progestin). The study also pointed out that women who eat carbohydrates when they are depressed or anxious are actually self-medicating their depression. Eating carbohydrates increases serotonin in the brain (the only problem is that it doesn't last long enough), so the addiction to sugar and carbs ensues. The study found that heavy consumption of refined carbohydrates, such as starches and sugars, have been connected to inflammation of the brain and linked directly to depression.

Ultimately, when you feed your body, you have to remember you are feeding your brain as well. The gray matter between your ears needs nutritional support for optimal thinking, focus, memory, and mood. Many of my patients that come to me with these kinds of mental problems find immediate relief when we balance their hormones, fix their diet and nutrient deficiencies, and ensure that they have proper absorption of nutrients via the gut. So fixing the body is often a surefire way of fixing the brain. Good news, we actually have some control over this.

Chronic stress takes a high toll on mental health. It affects your brain

18   James E. Gangwisch, Lorena Garcia, Lauren Hale, Dorothy S. Lane, M. Opler, Rebecca Rossom, Dolores Malaspina, and Martha Payne, "High Glycemic Index Diet as a Risk Factor for Depression: Analyses from the Women's Health Initiative," *American Journal of Clinical Nutrition* 102, no. 2 (2015), doi: 10.3945/ajcn.114.103846.

structure and function in an up-close-and-personal way. It accelerates brain aging, depletes beneficial neurotransmitters, increases fear, and halts the production of new brain cells while killing good ones already there. High stress increases the risk of psychiatric disorders; causes an inability to think, concentrate, and remember; and leaves you feeling depressed, low, anxious, and frantic. The positive news is that there are excellent ways to combat this while optimizing the new brain cell generation. So let's get to them. The following are the top seven dietary habits that adversely affect brain function and that you should avoid.

7 DIET HABITS THAT CAUSE A BRAIN AND MOOD SCRAMBLE

....

1. **Lack of omega-3 fats.** Lack of omega-3 fats causes brain damage. Seriously. Omega-3 fats form the basic structure of all of our cell membranes. Each brain cell is connected to other brain cells through about 40,000 synapses, and it takes a healthy cell to communicate appropriately, which means omega-3 and other healthy fats are needed to make a cell healthy. The fact is that the brain is mostly fat, which is why we need good fats to make our brain function optimal. They are hands-down the most important supplement for a healthy brain. The key here is omega-3 (not so much omega-6). Low levels of omega-3 fats have been linked to everything from depression to bipolar disease and dementia. The bad news is that bad fats (trans fats) kill cells' membranes and make them rigid, affecting their communication and slowing down the entire synapse. Consider eating brain-nourishing good fats such as:

   * Cold water fish, salmon, herring, cod, sable

- Omega-3 eggs
- Olive oil
- Omega-3 supplements
- Unrefined sesame oil
- Flax, hemp, nuts, and seeds

2. **Insufficient protein in the diet.** Proteins are messengers for the brain, and if you want a message relayed in your brain, you better have protein on board. Proteins are formed by eight essential amino acids that we get from our diet. These amino acids are necessary in making our brain's neurotransmitters, which keep us emotionally and mentally balanced. If you don't eat an adequate amount of protein at each meal, your brain is not going to work properly. You will feel sluggish, emotionally distraught, foggy, and depressed. Tryptophan is the main ingredient in making serotonin, the happy brain chemical. Tryptophan is present in most protein sources. No tryptophan means no serotonin, which means increased depression and anxiety. It's that simple.

3. **A high sugar, starch, carb diet.** I can't tell you how many thousands of patients have been cured from depression, obesity, anxiety, ADD, and other mood disorders by learning this one trick. *Stop the sugar-carb addiction.* To illustrate this, women will often feel overly undone with stress, which also means they probably have low blood sugar. This, in turn, creates the deep-seeded craving for carbs and simple sugars, a quick fix. But this is only a temporary fix, as the blast upward in blood glucose will come down just as quickly, leaving you feeling like you need another hit to keep going. What's really happening here is that carbohydrates or those treats laced with delicious sugar will effectively raise your serotonin and dopamine levels, creating a feeling of awe-someness (for just a bit) till it all collapses. When these levels drop, you will feel tired and will likely have a headache. You'll feel dizzy or nause-ated or you will ravenously crave more junk, making you irritable. The roller coaster of serotonin and dopamine swings are no fun, and frankly,

they make you feel half crazy after several rounds in a day. The strange thing to me is that some women go their entire life and never make this connection. I mean, I know ice cream is delicious, but . . .

4. **Instability in Blood.** The rise and fall of glucose in the blood sends off stress signals in your system, which then creates even more of a crisis and worsens the state of your brain balance. When glucose rises, so does insulin, which is inflammatory and not healthy in any way. It creates more belly fat, causes depression, leads to fatigue and irritability, and in no time will have you craving more. Eating high-glycemic foods or pushing your body beyond its blood sugar limits will deplete essential brain chemicals to the point that you have mood swings, headaches, and often anxiety. The chasing of the blood sugar and insulin levels is inflammatory to the brain and is toxic in many ways.

5. **Low Magnesium in the Diet.** The very foods, drinks, or drugs we are taking may be depleting your system of magnesium. Magnesium is essential in making serotonin and keeping you happy. Drinking alcohol regularly, eating high-sugar or processed foods, or taking certain medications can deplete your system of magnesium, creating low-level anxiety and depression.

6. **Lack of Good Carbohydrates:** While we have become something of a low-carb nation (or at least are trying to be), we need *good* carbs for optimal brain function. You should be reaching for real, whole, nourishing, plant-based carbohydrates. Some of these sources include vegetables, fruits, beans, nuts, and seeds. Plant-based carbohydrates contain the vitamins and nutrients you need to optimize brain chemicals (along with protein and good fats). They also contain fiber, which slows the release of sugar into the bloodstream, is excellent for digestion, and prevents the abrupt rise in insulin that goes along with it. In addition, colorful veggies and good carbs contain antioxidants that will nourish your brain.

7. **Nutrient-Deficient Diets:** The bottom line is that you need vitamins and nutrients to combat all the unhealthy things you encounter every

day. I am often told by women, "I eat great. I don't think I need vitamins or minerals." I chuckle and tell them that they probably don't need to take vitamins or be infused with nutrients and minerals if they are eating a perfectly clean, highly nutritious diet that comes from perfectly organic, nutrient-rich soils—not flown in or driven in thousands of miles or exposed to chemicals, pesticides, or antibiotics—and is not genetically modified, is organic, and is in its whole, untreated form. In addition, they have minimal stress, don't take medications that rob them of essential vitamins and minerals, only breathe in pure, non-polluted air, and take perfectly good care of themselves by sleeping, managing their stress, and not overdoing it with their workloads. (Then I take a deep breath because that was a mouthful, and I chuckle again.) This scenario would never exist. We need to give our bodies back what they need to make up for our muddied environment and lifestyle. Vitamin D, B complex, C, zinc, calcium, magnesium, selenium, folate, and essential fatty acids are only a few that we have to keep up on to feed our brain what it needs to stay balanced. These can be taken as supplements or given as an IV or in a shot.

FAST-TRACK TREATMENT FOR BRAIN BALANCE

So now it's time to start the quick treatment plan for a better brain. In one week, you'll be happy you did. Follow these simple steps, and I know you will find success!

- Take the full Brain Chemistry Quiz on my website (NishaJackson. com) to determine which of your neurochemicals are low. Dr. Julia Ross (who has been of tremendous support in my practice for many years now) developed this questionnaire to help determine what neurotransmitters you could be low in and what supplements you could use to create better balance and mood. You can also begin amino acid supplements to support the neurochemicals that are suffering.

- Immediately change your diet. Start eating the following foods for at least 80 percent of your weekly meals.

  - Food from the ground: veggies, fruits, avocados, sprouted grains

  - Foods that walk around: organic beef, turkey, chicken, eggs

  - Food from the sea: mercury-free fish, salmon, herring, and halibut

  - Nuts and seeds: pumpkin or flax seeds, almonds, walnuts, and macadamia nuts

- Stop eating sugar and starchy high-glycemic junk foods, and know they are as addictive as heroin and trigger the same centers in the brain as other highly addictive drugs. Be mindful that this is a normal response the next time you find yourself downing an entire bag of your favorite junk food or chips and can't pull yourself away from it. The best thing to do is not have it around.

- Begin taking vitamins that nourish the brain, including the following:

  - Omega-3 fatty acids

  - B complex (consider a B complex shot or nutrient IV)

  - Vitamin D (take this year-round and get your level tested)

  - Selenium (needed for optimal brain function)

  - Magnesium

- Consider herbs for added support to the brain, especially *ginkgo biloba*. Studies have shown that this herb helps promote oxygen to the brain and improves memory and performance.

- Consider using a small amount of dark chocolate (1 oz.) in the afternoon to boost dopamine instead of hitting the afternoon slump or snacking in the evening. This will help keep your levels optimal to avoid the sugar highs and lows.

- Take a time out. Stop working, stop looking at your phone, stop talking on the phone, stop surfing the web, stop listening to negative people, and stop filling your brain with things you can't change (like listening, reading, or watching the news). Give your brain a break. Even walking outside for ten minutes twice daily to regroup will do your brain a world of good.

- Go walk in nature. Getting outside is healing to the brain and the soul (and don't take your phone). Simply walk and let yourself feel what it is like to breathe and be silent, giving your entire system a reboot.

- Work your body. You get to work your brain every minute of every day. Think about what an imbalance this is for your brain. You need to sweat it out and let your brain become more nourished with a rich blood supply full of the oxygen it needs to operate smoothly.

- Balance your stress, thyroid, and ovarian hormones. Testosterone is so amazing for the brain. It is particularly important for focus, alertness, and a positive outlook on life, and it improves your ability to mentally manage stress. Your hormones and brain chemicals are constantly communicating with each other, and they need to stay in perfect balance to support the brain and its millions of daily tasks.

Brilliant Brain Balance Success Story

Jill was a 56-year-old go-getter. She worked ridiculous hours building her psychiatry business. She incorporated hormone balance and alternative therapy into her psychiatry practice and was super successful at it. She grew her company significantly in the previous six years and was my friend and colleague.

One day, she came to see me because she was worried sick that she could no longer remember names or recall events and was having intermittent anxiety. She had prided herself on taking the best care to eat, sleep, take supplements, and manage her hormones carefully for many years. But she had not paid attention to her workload and the brain overload that was troubling her. Because she was so busy, she had given up her outlet of riding horses and hiking and instead began racing into the crowded, loud gym to fit her spin class into her tight schedule. I asked her how many times she focused on only one thing at a time to recall the important events, and she knew that she was hypertasking on a crazy level and not paying attention or focusing anymore.

She took the brain quiz and was low in norepinephrine. This is not surprising because she was not sleeping deeply enough. She was also low in dopamine, which can affect focus and well-being. We ran a comprehensive hormone panel on her as well and discovered that she had very low cortisone and testosterone levels due to the extreme stress she was dealing with. After collecting all the information, we were ready to deal with the root cause of her issues rather than just treating her symptoms, and Jill was more than eager to get started.

Her game plan included the following:

• Immediately starting an amino acid replacement plan

• Optimizing her cortisol levels

- Optimizing her testosterone levels

- Finding a better work-life balance by delegating tasks and saying no to projects she didn't truly need or want to take on

- Undertaking more self-care by engaging in her hobbies and quiet periods of mindfulness

Jill undertook this journey with amazing fervor, and her turnaround was astounding. Within a month of having her hormones optimized and her brain supported, she was having no trouble with memory problems, she was happier, and she felt physically better than she had in years. Ultimately, she was most relieved that she was not entering dementia. She had simply lost track of where she was and how she got there.

She kept the momentum going too, and soon after this, she got a better balance in her workload and forced herself to fit in horseback riding and hiking to clear her brain (without her cell phone). She found out the hard way how important getting out into nature is for her to stay in the game with the best brain possible. Jill completely turned it around, and you can too. You just need to have your game plan and take it one step at a time. I believe in you.

6

Brilliant . . . but Feeling Fat: Everything You Need to Know about Stress and Belly Fat

"Those who think they have no time for healthy eating will sooner or later have to find time for illness."

—*EDWARD STANLEY*

In this chapter, we're going to examine how stress affects weight gain. But first things first: take this quiz to find out if you are insulin resistant.

QUIZ: ARE YOU INSULIN RESISTANT?

1. Do you feel hungry and shaky two to three hours after a meal? Y/N
2. If you miss a meal, do you feel irritable or tired? Y/N
3. Do you tend to retain water after eating salty foods? Y/N

4. Do you get tired a few hours after eating? Y/N

5. Has anyone in your immediate family by blood (not spouse or in-laws) had diabetes or hypoglycemia? Y/N

6. Has anyone in your family had heart disease, polycystic ovary syndrome, or gout? Y/N

7. Is most of your excess weight carried around your middle/abdomen? Y/N

8. Do you tend to gain weight quickly or have a hard time losing on any diet? Y/N

9. Do you experience frequent food cravings for sugary or starchy foods? Y/N

10. Do you suffer from mood swings? Y/N

11. Are you usually tired or fatigued in afternoon or early evening? Y/N

12. Do you find it difficult to lose weight on a low-fat diet? (Answer no if you haven't tried a low-fat diet.) Y/N

13. Do you have mood swings or PMS? Y/N

14. Do your food cravings, especially for sweet or starchy foods, occur in the late afternoon or evening? Y/N

15. Have you experienced weight loss, excessive thirst, or frequent urination? Y/N

If you answered yes to more than five of the above questions, you are likely suffering from unstable insulin production in response to the foods you are eating. This is what's causing you to gain weight around your belly and why you've probably had such a hard time losing it. Fortunately, now you know what's going on, and there are ways to treat insulin resistance. But first, let's talk about where this condition comes from.

If you find yourself storing more fat around the middle than you would like, and the quick-fix tricks you have used to get rid of it are no longer working, it is possible that you are insulin resistant. The good news is that it can be treated if you attack it the correct way. And in case the running theme of the book didn't give it away already, this is all tied into your stress.

THE STRESS-WEIGHT GAIN-BELLY FAT CONNECTION

While high levels of stress may be unavoidable at times, the intense and chronic state of stress could be making you store fat at an accelerated rate, especially around your midsection. Even if you try to eat well and exercise, chronic high stress can prevent you from losing this weight. Here's a breakdown of what happens: First, remember that your body responds to all stress in exactly the same way. So, every time you have a stressful day, your brain instructs your cells to release potent hormones. You get a burst of adrenaline, which taps stored energy so you can fight or flee. At the same time, you get a surge of cortisol, which tells your body to replenish that energy even though you haven't used very many calories. This can make you hungry… *very* hungry. And your body will keep on pumping out cortisol as long as the stress continues. Finally, the cortisol interacts with insulin (a fat-storage hormone), putting your body into the dreaded fat storage zone, increasing your cravings and appetite all at the same time. Talk about hitting a girl when she's down.

Few of us reach for carrots in these situations. Instead, we crave sweet, salty, and high-fat foods, because they stimulate the brain to release pleasure chemicals that reduce tension. This soothing effect becomes addicting, so every time you're anxious, you want fattening, sugary foods, because they do the trick.

With your adrenal glands pumping out cortisol, production of the muscle-building hormone testosterone slows down. Over time, this drop causes a decrease in your muscle mass, so you burn fewer calories, even at rest. This occurs naturally as you age, but high cortisol levels accelerate the process. Cortisol also encourages your body to store fat—especially belly (visceral) fat, which is particularly dangerous because it surrounds vital organs and releases fatty acids into your blood, raising cholesterol and insulin levels and paving the way for heart disease and diabetes.

You may be thinking, *What's* visceral *fat? Isn't fat just fat?* Not exactly. Your body contains two different types of fat: subcutaneous fat and visceral fat. Subcutaneous fat is the fat you can pinch in your nephew's cheeks or at your belly area. Whereas visceral fat is what builds up around your vital organs, wrapping itself around your heart, liver, and pancreas and settling in your belly, where it releases numerous toxins. The difference between these two types of fats explains why it's possible for someone to appear relatively thin but still be unhealthy due to the visceral fat that's stored deep inside their body.

If you have too much visceral fat, you are at a greater risk for the following:

- Diabetes

- Heart disease

- Certain cancers

- Alzheimer's disease

But how do you know if you have too much visceral fat? Although an MRI is the most accurate way to determine how much excess visceral fat you store, a much simpler (and less expensive) test is a simple waistline measurement. Simply put, because 10 percent of our total fat is normally stored as visceral fat, and visceral fat is stored near the abdominal cavity, a protruding belly is a pretty good indicator of too much visceral fat.

How Stressed-Out Women Pack on Belly Fat

Let's quickly break down what we've learned so far so we can make a couple of conclusions to build off on. Stress causes high levels of cortisol. High levels of cortisol cause your body to store more fat, known as visceral fat. Visceral fat is stored within your abdominal cavity, meaning—you guessed it—it can appear as belly fat. Not only does this happen, but when you're constantly flooding your body with cortisol, your appetite can increase and your desire for fatty foods may increase as well. Because of all these reasons, the conclusions we can make about losing belly fat are

1. It's about diet and exercise. What you eat and how much you move make a difference.

2. It's about managing stress. You have to stop the cycle putting you in "fat storage mode."

These are the biggest hurdles to losing belly fat, but they are well worth conquering, not only for your looks but also to keep you healthy and prevent disease and inflammation everywhere in your body and cells.

A study conducted at Yale University showed that stress causes excess abdominal fat in otherwise slender women.[19] It was the first study to show that lean, healthy women with abdominal fat have exaggerated responses to cortisol. They also found that women with greater abdominal fat had more negative moods, depression, and higher levels of life stress.

Why Late-Night Eating Reduces the Quality of Sleep

Humans are designed to burn fat through the night because it burns long and slow—in contrast to sugar and carbs, which burn quickly. When you eat breakfast, your body stops burning fat. Today, because of undetected blood sugar issues, many people never go into fat metabolism during the night at all. Instead, they attempt to burn sugar and carbs through the night as they did during the day. With sugar and short-chain carbs delivering only short, quick bursts of energy, sleeping through the night becomes an insurmountable task.

As the amount of sleep decreases, blood sugar increases, which only

---

19   Elissa S. Epel, Bruce McEwen, Teresa Seeman, Karen Matthews, Grace Castellazzo, Kelly D. Brownell, Jennifer Bell, and Jeannette R. Ickovics, "Stress and Body Shape: Stress-Induced Cortisol Secretion Is Consistently Greater Among Women with Central Fat," *Psychosomatic Medicine* 62, no. 5 (2000): 623–632, https://www.ncbi.nlm.nih.gov/pubmed/11020091.

escalates the issue. Lack of sleep has been shown to raise blood sugar levels, and this can dramatically increase the risk of diabetes. Higher blood sugar means less long-lasting fat metabolism in the night and even less sleep. See the cycle?

Researchers at Boston University School of Medicine found that people who slept less than six hours a night had far more blood sugar problems compared to those who got eight hours of sleep.[20] This illustrates that the cycle of sleep deprivation raises blood sugar, and unstable blood sugar, in turn, compromises quality sleep. But how does this vicious cycle even get started in the first place?

When you don't get enough sleep, you wake up tired and reach for that vanilla latte or cola, sending your blood sugar right back up. Without realizing it, cravings for energy drinks, bars, breads, pastas, and sweets become the norm. This constant surge of sugar and simple carbs puts significant strain on the pancreas. The result is a condition called *prediabetes*, which amazingly affects one-third of the American population. And, according to the CDC, 90 percent of those people don't even know they have it.

If you are looking to get better, deeper sleep and not be packing on the pounds, consider what is happening when you eat late at night.

Eating before bed or drinking right until bedtime (alcohol or sugary drinks) or snacking while watching TV might help you go to sleep, but the interruptions in sleeping will wreak havoc on your metabolism and leave you feeling unrested and needing more sleep the next morning. See the following graph to understand the rise and fall in glucose with eating/drinking late and how this affects the "wake-up hormone" cortisol (not so great to have this escalate at night).

---

20   Jack Challem and Ron Hunninghake, *Stop Prediabetes Now: The Ultimate Plan to Lose Weight and Prevent Diabetes* (Hoboken, New Jersey: John Wiley and Sons, 2009): 234.

Nighttime Cortisol Syndrome

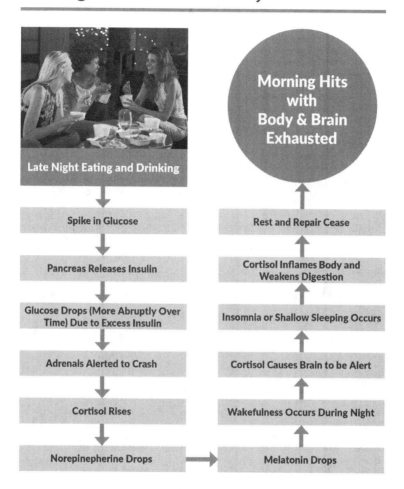

Figure 6.1: Nighttime Cortisol Syndrome

There is hope here, though, and it comes with such a simple change in our daily habits. I have found that many of my patients feel better when they stop eating early in the evening and do not eat until later the next morning. This increases the number of hours they are fasting at night.

By making this small shift in their eating patterns, my patients find they are able to lose weight, sleep better, and have less perceived stress. The question you should be asking now is… *Why?*

The Connection Between Late-Night Eating and Belly Fat

When you eat or drink late at night, especially if you're having foods that cause your glucose to rise (sugar, dairy, and starchy foods are the worst), you're going to set off a host of negative reactions in your body. And the higher the rise in glucose and insulin levels, the more profound the negative effects. Additionally, if you eat a meal and then continue to snack and drink throughout the evening, right up until bedtime, the insulin and glucose in your blood will continue to climb higher and higher each time. This not only makes your body continue to work to digest the food in the evening when you actually are needing fewer calories, it also puts you straight into the dreaded fat-storage zone.

This is common with people who love partying and eating dinner and dessert later at night, or who continue to snack right until bedtime. All of these common behaviors ramp up insulin production, creating more belly fat and causing you to get less restorative sleep (which, infuriatingly enough, also causes weight gain). While eating late at night can make you drowsy initially, it will also prolong digestion, which interrupts the process of restoration while sleeping, causing you to wake up feeling worse the next day. All this being said, it's best to eat your biggest meal before midafternoon and to then have a light evening meal of 500 calories or less. Include some chicken, extra-lean meat, or fish at dinner to help curb snack attacks in the middle of the night.

Why Reducing Calories Reduces the Stress Response

This strategy of increasing the amount of time between your last meal of one day and your first meal of the next is commonly referred to as *intermittent fasting* because you are creating periods of time in which your glucose and insulin levels get down to a fasting level each day. The reason intermittent fasting works so well is because there are two fuels your body can burn for energy: sugar and fat. And you have about six to eight hours of stored sugar as glycogen in your muscles and in your liver. Once you exhaust that, then you're out of fuel for the most part, unless your enzymes are adapted to burning fat.

Most people have plenty of fat to burn. The problem is when your glycogen stores are being consistently replenished by eating every six to eight hours, then the enzymes that are adapted to burn fat for energy get impaired, preventing your body from burning the fat. This creates a vicious cycle, which I think is exacerbated by having breakfast, as this doesn't allow your body to enter that glorious fat-burning zone. You need that 12-hour window (or more) where you're not eating any food, to upregulate your enzymes to burn fat, downregulate the enzymes to burn carbs, and shift your body into fat-burning mode as your primary way of supplying energy. There are three major benefits to accomplishing this:

1. Your hunger for junk food and sugars disappears. It's the closest thing to magic I've ever seen with respect to diet.

2. You're able to normalize your body fat.

3. Your weight typically goes down, unless you're very muscular (and it doesn't decrease your muscle mass—which by the way is an extra benefit).

BENEFITS OF INTERMITTENT FASTING

The benefits of intermittent fasting are a hot topic in the wellness world today, with research supporting its ability to decrease inflammation, lower insulin levels, heal the gut, and teach the body to use its fat for energy—instead of always relying on the food that you are eating. But most important of all is that there is good evidence that intermittent fasting can even increase the number of years you have to live. As a functional medicine practitioner, it's one of my favorite tools to use for my patients, because it works so well.

Fat-Storing and Hunger Hormones

The connection between fasting, hormones, and body weight is quite interesting. Let's go through a quick overview of this connection that could help you lose body fat and feel exceedingly better.

Apart from being a great way to control your weight, intermittent fasting is one of the best tools for treating hunger problems, slowed metabolism, and blood sugar issues that are negatively affecting your hormones. When my patients have high stress and are also packing on weight around their midsection, this is the first dietary change I make. I do this because it increases their metabolism and lowers their insulin levels all at once.

Another metabolism buster, however, that women can experience at any age is—leptin resistance. This is yet another hormonal problem created by stress that leads to weight gain and the inability to lose weight. Intermittent fasting has been shown to correct leptin resistance while reducing your appetite at the same time. Intermittent fasting has also been shown to positively affect the hunger hormone ghrelin. Amazingly, this can directly improve and support dopamine levels in the brain too, which creates a better sense of overall well-being and is the perfect example of the reality of the gut-brain axis connection.

Estrogen and Progesterone

Your brain and ovaries communicate through the brain-ovary axis, or hypothalamic-pituitary-gonadal (HPG) axis. Your brain sends hormones to your ovaries to signal them to release estrogen and progesterone. If your HPG axis isn't working (as is often the case with high stress), it can affect your overall health, mood, menstrual cycles, and metabolism.

Women are usually more sensitive to the effects of intermittent fasting. This is due to the fact that women have more kisspeptin, which creates greater sensitivity to fasting. This means their cycle can temporarily be altered as they are losing body fat. This is normal and common, and it shows you the connection between weight changes and female hormones. Ultimately, this is a diet that I would suggest everyone give a try, as studies continue to show that intermittent fasting supports female hormones and corrects insulin resistance, which cause a myriad of health problems for women of any age.[21]

Intermittent Fasting Options

The following are some ways you can fast intermittently. Choose the plan that works best for you, and stick with it for optimal results.

1. Try a modified fast, two nonconsecutive days a week (such as Sunday and Thursday). This means on these days you would eat 500–750 calories early in the day with your last food at 6:00 p.m. to 7:00 p.m. For best results, do only light exercise on the two fasting days per week and eat clean (low sugar/flour/starch) on all other days of the week.

2. Try basic nighttime fasting. Fast from 12 to 15 hours at night at least five nights per week. This means you could stop eating at 6:00 p.m. to 7:00 p.m. and then not eat the next day until 9:00 or 10:00 am. Drinking filtered water and unsweetened herbal teas are totally fine during this period.

---

21 Mark P. Mattson and Ruiqian Wan, "Beneficial Effects of Intermittent Fasting and Caloric Restriction on the Cardiovascular and Cerebrovascular Systems," *Journal of Nutritional Biochemistry* 16, no. 3 (2005): 129–137, doi: 10.1016/j.jnutbio.2004.12.007.

3. Engage in nighttime extended fasting. With extended nighttime fasting, you will fast at night for 16–17 hours, two to three times per week, or every other day. For best results, stop eating at 6:00 p.m. and do not eat again until 11:00 a.m.–noon the next day. As with basic fasting, water and unsweetened herbal teas are fine to consume during the fasting hours.

4. Experiment with a limited daytime eating option. Consider consuming your food between 9:00 a.m. and 6:00 p.m. every day.

5. Try a weekday fasting option. With this option, try eating between noon and 6:00 p.m. Monday through Thursday weekly. Drink a good antioxidant-rich tea during the morning hours to help.

6. Or you can try an every-other-day plan. For a more aggressive approach, drop your caloric intake to between 500 and 750 calories every other day and then practice clean eating (veggies, proteins, nuts, seeds, fruit, and whole unprocessed foods) on the alternate days.

Whichever plan you choose, consider adding these days gradually in the beginning to limit the side effects of hunger. If you have health challenges, consider discussing this with your nutritionist or medical practitioner first. Listen to your body as it tells you how you are feeling, and know that you *will* be hungry and your stomach *will* be shrinking (which is a good thing). This feeling will fade over time; you just have to stick with it. Until this happens, I would suggest you think about embracing the feeling of hunger and listening to your body. Most people have no idea what real hunger feels like. And most women are scared to death of feeling hungry and are worried sick they will have a drop in glucose.

While you do need to pay attention to the signals your body is sending you, I think we have taken the idea of low blood sugar a little too far. Most of us have enough carbs stored in our livers to last quite a while without feeling weak. The key is not to overdo it initially as you are starting to increase the number of hours of nighttime fasting. Instead, take it gradually, and try to increase the number of fasting hours over time as you make this part of your normal routine. I also recommend adding 4–8 grams of branched-chain amino acid (BCAA) supplements, which come in powder and capsule form. These can help improve the positive impact of fasting and help take the edge off of mood-related fasting issues.

CANDIDA: THE SCOURGE TO FAT LOSS HIDING IN YOUR GUT

Gut health has gone from a niche interest to something that is widely acknowledged as crucial to vitality and well-being. *Candida overgrowth* is the common term used for an overgrowth of the yeast *Candida albicans*, a condition also known as a candida imbalance. Under normal circumstances, and in the body of healthy individuals, *Candida albicans* will pose no threat; it is simply one of the many microbes that live in the body's digestive tract, mouth, vagina, and even moist areas of the skin. The problem is that candida is always on the lookout for a way to multiply, and it will jump at the first opportunity to do so. It is also clever and will build "forts" (biofilms) around communities of candida to keep them safe. If the other bacteria and microbes that live in your body are unable to keep candida in check, you will quickly have an overgrowth and a host of uncomfortable symptoms to go with it. An imbalanced gut flora is not just an inconvenience—it's a serious malfunction that can have consequences in multiple areas of your body.

Candida can be responsible for excess fat deposits, and in order to lose this weight, you need to treat the root cause—the underlying candida infection. Candida thrives on sugar, its preferred source of fuel. When you are in the throes of a candida infestation, the candida will cause you to crave carbs and sugar in all its forms. Maintaining a healthy metabolism—the key to maintaining a healthy weight—is impossible when you need to feed a sugar-craving organism like candida. It's like being pregnant with a baby that never comes to term and doesn't make your skin glow.

Worse yet, candida toxins also overload the liver and release different toxins into your bloodstream as candida cells naturally die off. This is part of the natural life cycle of the organism. The toxins that are constantly being released need to be processed by your liver. But your liver can quickly become overworked. To cope, your liver will store toxins to be processed at a later date. But where does it store those toxins? In your fat cells. That's right; we've come full circle. The candida toxins will show up as stubborn weight around your abdomen, hips, and thighs.

Symptoms of candida overgrowth include the following:

- Toenail fungus

- Vaginal thrush

- Fatigue

- Headaches

- Anxiety

- Rectal itching

- Hormonal imbalances

- Digestive issues

- Mood swings

- Dizziness

- Sore throat

- Oral thrush

- Persistent cough

- Leaky gut

- Skin rashes

- Acne

- Brain fog

- Bladder infections

- Low sex drive

- Sinus inflammation

- Allergies

- Sugar cravings

Diagnosing and Treating Systemic Candida

Systemic candida is a problem that is currently affecting more women than ever. The following are the top three ways to diagnose this condition:

1. **Comprehensive stool analysis:** Although not fun, this test can, in fact, reliably determine the levels of *Candida albicans* in your gut and let you know if they are abnormal.

2. **Candida antibodies test:** This handy test determines if your immune system has created antibodies as a response to fight a candida infection. Three different types of antibodies can indicate an overgrowth of candida. The antibodies that can be tested with a blood test are IgG, IgA, and IgM antibodies.

3. **Written test:** There also is a written test for diagnosing candida you can take. (Visit my website, NishaJackson.com, to take the Candida Test.) If you score above 140 on this test, then you most likely have an overgrowth of candida in your gut.

The best way to rebalance your gut is to take a high-potency probiotic. These can be taken as a supplement, or they can come from foods like kefir and yogurt (or ideally, both). Other dietary and lifestyle changes will also help to restore balance to your gut. Some of these changes include

- Reducing your stress levels

- Cutting back on your caffeine intake

- Eliminating added sugars from your diet

Antifungal foods and supplements such as oregano, garlic, grape seed extract, apple cider vinegar, caprylic acid, coconut oil, and high-potency probiotics can also be helpful in weakening an overgrowth of pathogenic yeasts like candida, while restoring the gut balance. The use of antifungal medications, such as fluconazole and nystatin, is effective for treating candida, and they are often used for longer periods of time—up to six weeks. They have been shown to be especially effective when paired with a restricted diet that eliminates sugar, flour, and processed foods.

WHAT IS POLYCYSTIC OVARIAN SYNDROME?

This is a big issue for women struggling with their weight. If you've been diagnosed with polycystic ovary syndrome, or PCOS, the numbers on the scale may seem to tick up no matter what you do—almost as if just looking at food makes you gain weight. PCOS is known to be a metabolic disorder, wreaking havoc on your body's ability to burn calories. It also makes our bodies insulin resistant and more susceptible to storing fat.

With PCOS, the problems women experience can stem from cysts in the ovaries or adrenal (stress induced) dysfunction, both of which are most likely connected to the delicate balance between brain, adrenal, and ovarian hormones being ransacked with stress. This leads to over-production or insensitivity of insulin, which then starts a cascade of massive hormone disruption. Women with PCOS will typically produce higher levels of testosterone, DHEA, insulin, and estrogen, and they will underproduce progesterone because of a lack of ovulation.

Excess testosterone is linked to higher rates of insulin resistance, acne, facial hair growth, irregular bleeding, and male-pattern baldness. When fat percentages rise, your insulin resistance and production can increase further (since fat cells produce insulin). This vicious cycle can lead to diabetes and infertility, as the high insulin impairs women's ability to ovulate and produce progesterone. Lack of progesterone creates depression, anxiety, and mood changes linked to PMS, painful or missed periods, and insomnia.

Estrogen dominance creates a fat storage state and leads to PMS, menstrual problems, and mood swings. The worst part is that this entire complex of hormone imbalance often goes undetected and can make you pack on weight like never before. Excess insulin production leads to insulin resistance, which in turn decreases your ability to use insulin effectively. When the body cannot use insulin properly, it secretes more insulin to make glucose available to cells. The resulting excess insulin is thought to additionally boost androgen production by the ovaries, truly bringing the hormone imbalances full circle.

How Is PCOS Linked to Stress?

Here's the confusing concept: Some women can have normally functioning ovaries with no cysts and no insulin resistance yet still fit the
symptomatic profile of PCOS. This means some women gain weight, have
symptoms of higher testosterone, and yet do not exhibit the normal profile of PCOS. The brain is heavily involved with the output of androgenic
(male-like) hormone production, and the adrenals are also responsible for
PCOS symptoms in some women. This is newer information, and most
medical doctors still do not realize that a subset of women have PCOS
simply from high ongoing stress and do not fit the traditional clinical
picture of PCOS.

When women are exposed to extreme chronic stress, they will often
have elevated DHEA levels in response to the brain signals of ACTH.
This is the brain's way of trying to protect the body from the long-term
effects of chronic stress, but ultimately this leads to more weight gain,
erratic periods, mood changes, hair loss, facial hair, acne, or skin problems, which are all associated with PCOS. If PCOS is neglected, undiagnosed, or not treated properly, it can be a precursor to a variety of serious
health conditions, including heart disease, liver and kidney disorders,
breast cancer, obesity, diabetes, infertility, and possibly Alzheimer's disease and premature aging.

How to Diagnose and Treat PCOS

PCOS is diagnosed through blood testing of the hormone levels, evaluation of the current symptoms, and ultrasound to look for possible cysts
lining the periphery of the ovaries. The treatment of PCOS is often a
combination of treatments, including massive overhaul of the diet to a
low-glycemic-index regimen. Hormonal changes include lowering testosterone with medications, herbs, and in some cases birth control pills
or the use of a mild diuretic called spironolactone. Insulin is lowered

through a strict low-sugar, low-carbohydrate diet; exercise (cardio); the use of a medication called metformin; and/or a supplement called chromium picolinate. Progesterone is optimized with the use of bioidentical progesterone, which immediately supports the mood, lowers anxiety, reduces stress, and helps regulate menstrual cycles and periods while promoting weight loss.

Losing weight with even a 10 percent body fat loss can lower insulin and androgen levels immediately. This will also help restore ovulation and fertility for women. Untreated PCOS can also significantly increase a woman's risk of developing diabetes and infertility. In addition, untreated or undiagnosed PCOS is linked to high blood pressure, sleep apnea, abnormal uterine bleeding, cholesterol abnormalities, metabolic syndrome, heart disease, uterine and breast cancer, obesity, menstrual problems, heavy bleeding, and complicated pregnancies. If we can diagnose and treat PCOS early, we can reduce the risk of these long-term complications.

FAST TRACK: TAKING YOUR PLAN ON THE GO

So now that you have a better picture of how stress interacts with every part of your metabolism and your body's ability to burn calories, I want to give you some quick options for getting into a fat-burning zone and out of a fat-storage zone. This is *the* Belly Fat Blast. Here we go.

- Meditate. If you don't currently have a meditation practice in place, now is the time to develop one. Even five minutes of meditation, where you focus on your breath and sit calmly, will help reduce your body's response to stress, which ultimately will help control insulin and glucose swings. (Plus, it will downregulate your nervous system, which will slow down cravings and appetite.)

- Consider starting one of the intermittent fasting plans that are listed in this chapter, increase your fasting hours and days as your body feels able. Too many calories are a problem as you age. The bottom line is that you have to stop eating so much. It's a numbers game, and eating fewer calories will improve your energy, lower your weight, and increase your metabolism. Added benefits are better sleep as well as improved digestion and mental functioning. You need to know what you are taking in and burning off during the day to make strides with weight loss and improved health.

- Lower the starchy comfort foods in your diet. Stop kidding yourself that going gluten-free is healthy eating. Instead, you must look at the total number of carbs you are eating. Just because something is gluten free doesn't mean that it doesn't make your glucose and insulin soar, leading to increased belly fat and fatigue. Count the carbs you are eating and try to make the most of them. Eat mostly vegetables, and aim for high fiber and the lowest sugar possible in the carbs you eat. This is where it's so important to read your labels: four grams of sugar = one *teaspoon* of sugar! For instance, mocha drinks have 40 grams of sugar, which equals 10 teaspoons of sugar. Wow! And, most importantly, do not eat excessive carbs during the day. This will slow your weight loss down and slow you down physically. Instead, focus your diet on proteins, veggies, and good fats.

- Drink ten eight-ounce glasses of water with lemon squeezed in it daily. This will support your liver in the fat detoxification process.

- Eat one gram of protein daily for every pound of body weight until your weight loss normalizes. This will stabilize your glucose and help you be less hungry. Protein also contains amino acids, which support brain chemicals, helping you have less anxiety, mood-eating, and cravings. Protein deficiency will leave you hungry, nervous, irritable, moody, depressed, sluggish, and mentally foggy. Not including protein with each meal will often result in craving sweets and will keep you from getting from one meal to the next without fading out. Your body will retain water, and you will more easily gain weight through the action of insulin.

- Consider the cleansing diet (see Appendix H) for the next two weeks to help jump-start your weight loss and grant you better glucose/insulin control. This diet is one I have been using in my practice for 25 years now (because it works so well). It is the best hormonal-stress control diet I have found, and it has the added benefit that it also takes the fat right off your belly. Just remember that it's time for you to reduce the excessive carbohydrates. As we age, and certainly with high stress, we do not need as many quick carbs in our diet because, let's face it, we are not running a marathon today. So, in order for our body to stay tuned for optimal metabolism, we need to lower our intake of the foods that cause insulin (the belly fat hormone) to rise. It helps to have less than two starch servings per day, and some days go without them altogether. Furthermore, consider getting your carbohydrates from veggies.

- Eat dark chocolate later in the afternoon. Consuming just one ounce will raise serotonin and calm your nervous system, helping you calm yourself before you go home and literally raid the refrigerator or, worse yet, eat an entire dinner *while* you are fixing dinner (not good for the waistline!).

- Begin focusing on your breath as a way to control your cortisol production and stress. Every time you go to the bathroom, sit there and take five slow, deep breaths in and hold for the count of five and then exhale to the count of seven, blowing all your air out. If you find yourself really stressed, do five more deep cleansing breaths.

- Exercise and move your body every day to the point of being out of breath. I don't care what you do for exercise, but you better be moving your body somehow, some way—no excuses (not even the weather). Aim for ten minutes twice a day and work up to 45 minutes of briskly working out. Now listen to me: If you make the fatal decision to *not* move your body and sweat during the week, you will eventually be tired, depressed, fat, and your body and face will age at an accelerated rate. In addition, our stressful lives constantly tap our brain and nervous system, leaving us with a terrible imbalance between our bodies and our brain, which makes us feel as if we can't handle the stress. This is why we end up drinking alcohol, eating poorly, and habituating to all sorts of unhealthy behaviors. Bottom line: Exercising five days a week or more gets you the results you need, and that is one hot body!

· Drop down and give me ten! Start using simple, quick muscle-building and firming exercises to tone your body and stay healthy. Start with a simple full-body plan. In our late thirties, we women begin to lose up to 3 percent of our muscle mass each year. Yikes! If you wonder why your metabolism is in the tank, there's your answer. Fortunately, there is an easy solution to stop the muscle loss: Start simply by doing sit-ups, push-ups (modified are fine), and lunges, and work up to as many as you can each day, even if you have to start with only a few. Going to the gym and getting some professional direction or even purchasing exercise bands and doing a full-body workout three days a week for 20 minutes will do you wonders for how toned you look, and will help prevent the appearance of saggy skin as you age. (Plus, who doesn't want to maintain strength and flexibility as they age?)

· Do 25 push-ups to start, and work up to 90 push-ups: three sets of 30, three to four days a week, with a quick rest in between (you can do women's style, men's style, military style, or on an exercise ball, which is my favorite).

- Do 25 lunges, keeping your knee almost touching the ground as you lunge: start easy and work up to 90 deep lunges, rotating legs, three to four days a week.

- Do 25 belly crunches to start, and work up 100 or more with short, slow movements up and back (partially up), focusing on the belly button tightening. Do this on an exercise ball or the floor. Try to do this three to four days per week, but go slowly and try to increase your numbers each week. Feel the burn! It's your stomach tightening.

- Get your hormones checked, and make sure that you are not low in thyroid hormone, testosterone, or progesterone, which can all cause weight gain. Ensure that your balance of estrogen to progesterone is normal and that you have optimal levels of glucose and insulin.

- Consider testing for candida. If you test positive, seek treatment to optimize the gut balance and improve your digestion and absorption of your important vitamins, nutrients, and minerals. For some, this is imperative for weight loss and better energy, and should not be ignored.

- Do the Cleansing Jump-start Diet for Fat Loss on Adrenal Reset (as outlined in Appendix H).

- Take supplements to control your appetite and cravings (see Appendix E):

  - Mood supplement with 5HTP and GABA—to reduce cravings and mood eating

  - Chromium picolinate to lower insulin—three times per day 200–400mcg

- Stress support/adrenal supplements to enhance focus and energy and improve your ability to stay on track

- Lipotropics MIC shots or tablets for weight loss—to improve the liver's ability to metabolize fat

- Craving supplement—this will help raise norepinephrine, which reduces cravings due to mood

Fat Blast Success Story

Kacey was an RN living in Dallas who had an impossible time finding hormone help where she lived, so she asked me to do a series of live-web consults and treatments with her. Kacey had a long history of being a strong athlete and was always at the top of her game in everything she did. She had two children later in life, was the manager of a level-one trauma unit, on the board at her kids' school, was an accomplished artist on the side, and had never really struggled with her weight before. In the past year, however, her weight had ballooned up 40 pounds. She had been seen by several medical doctors, who all told her she was normal and that she just needed to be careful with her intake of calories. As you can imagine, this was not very helpful, and she was frustrated and tearful during the consults, saying she hated her body and that it was affecting her confidence and her relationship with her husband. She tried to follow a low-carb diet but would end up eating everything in sight.

I knew I could help Kacey, and luckily, as a nurse, she had access to my usual hormone testing. The lab reports showed low cortisol, progesterone, vitamin D, and B12; and high testosterone, DHEA, insulin, and glucose. She also had low serotonin, dopamine, and pregnenolone. Additionally, she tested positive for Hashimoto's thyroiditis and had a very low T3 level (active thyroid). She had a perfect storm of issues that were going to be complicated for her to tackle, but I knew that I could help get her confidence and her life back!

Her game plan included the following:

- Immediately fixing all of her hormone levels with bioidentical hormones

- Starting medication to lower testosterone and insulin levels

- Starting supplements to fix her low vitamin levels

- Starting an intermittent fasting plan supplemented with a low-glycemic diet

- Lowering her stress by unloading some of the tasks she could put on hold

- Working on equipping her body to better manage stress with regular exercise and mindfulness training

- Starting on weight loss supplements during her journey to get back in shape

Kacey was a determined woman, and by carefully following her game plan, she started seeing results almost immediately. Within six months, she had lost 46 pounds. More importantly, she felt great physically and emotionally.

She checks in with me yearly now to ensure her levels are normal and says she has to constantly watch herself with stress, as her natural tendency is to take on too much. But she knows that doing too much is the quickest way to end up in the situation she desperately doesn't want to be in—again. She says no more often to excess work and yes more often to the things she loves and that are good for her. She has become one of the best advocates for health I know, which, ultimately, is what this is all about.

7

Don't Be Moody; Shake Your Booty!: How to Move Your Body for Stress Relief, Beauty, Energy, and Fat Loss!

"In order to kick ass, you must first lift your foot."
— JEN SINCERO

We're going to explore the connection between exercise, energy levels, fat loss, and stress relief. Spend a moment with the following quiz to assess your level of fitness.

QUIZ: HOW FIT ARE YOU?

Answer yes or no to the following fitness scenarios:

1. Can you hold a plank for at least 60 seconds? Y/N
2. Can you do 27 push-ups in a minute? Y/N

3. Can you easily walk up five flights of stairs without stopping? Y/N

4. Can you get up from sitting on the ground with no assistance? Y/N

5. Can you hold a wall sit for over a minute? Y/N

6. Do you incorporate a cardio workout into your routine at least three days per week? Y/N

7. Can you do more than 60 crunches in one minute? Y/N

8. Can you fast walk, jog, or run two miles without stopping? Y/N

9. Can you do 20 lunges without stopping? Y/N

10. Can you touch your toes easily? Y/N

11. Is your BMI under 25? Y/N

....

If you answered yes to only 1–3 of the above questions, you are, to put it nicely, in less than optimal shape.

If you said yes to 4–8 of the above questions, you are in moderate shape. Your consolation prize: You get to learn how to say yes to the rest of the questions!

If you said yes to 9–11 of the above questions, congratulations—you are in good shape (but hey, don't get cocky—keep reading).

NO EXCUSES

When I started my medical practice 25 years ago, I had a license plate that said *NOEXCUSES*, which was kind of my motto at the time. And though that car and its license plate are long gone, I still try to apply this kind of mentality to everything I do. It has served to keep me on track in all areas of my life. I think excuses are disabling.

Over the past two decades of working with highly successful and powerful women, I have found that there is one thing they make excuses for more than anything else. The thing they let go of that would help them stay balanced and sane the most: *exercise*. When we are experiencing excessive stress, we tend to abandon exercise. Excuses like "I have no time," "My body hurts," "It's dark and cold," "I don't have time to get to the gym," "I hate going to the gym," "I can't sleep at night," "I can't get up in the morning," "I am not motivated," "I'm exhausted," and "Exercise doesn't even make a difference with my weight" prevail over their better impulses.

The reality is that you will be *way* more stressed, depressed, and out of balance when you are *not* moving your body, so there should be no excuse for you to want to feel like this. Moving your body must be part of your routine for you to stay sharp, be positive, act confident, age better, look better, and be strong. Most important of all, exercise provides an outlet for stress to get out of your body.

HOW EXERCISE SUPPORTS THE BRAIN

There are too many advantages of exercise to list in this short chapter, but the big ones are reducing the odds of heart disease, stroke, obesity, diabetes, depression, and dementia. And the way that exercise can protect the brain is phenomenal. I want to touch on this because, let's face it, without our brilliant brains, we would be lost.

Exercise and regular movement of the body has been found to clear up brain fog, heal the brain, grow new brain cells, and reduce the negative effects of aging on the brain. Even more amazingly, regular aerobic exercise—the kind that gets your heart pumping and sweat glands working—appears to boost the size of your hippocampus, the tiny area of the brain that is involved with memory, the ability to think, and learning new things.

With dementia on the rise, and one new case of it diagnosed every three seconds globally,[22] it's time to incorporate some brain protection

---

22 "10 Facts on Dementia," World Health Organization, accessed October 25, 2018, http://www.who.int/features/factfiles/dementia/dementia_facts/en/index2.html.

measures into our daily plan. Exercise promotes memory and clear thinking in several ways. And, for brilliant women, the most important of these is that it reduces inflammation and stimulates growth factors (chemicals in the brain that support the health of brain cells, growth of new blood vessels, and even more new brain cells). Exercise also improves mood (dramatically) and is one of the best ways to treat depression and anxiety. Finally, moving our body daily helps improve sleep cycles, which we now know protect our brains in ways unmatched by any other supplement or preventive measure.

If none of that has convinced you to start exercising, how about this: Studies have shown that people who exercise have bigger brains.[23] The areas of the brain also involved with thinking and memory—the prefrontal cortex and medial temporal cortex—have a larger volume in people who move their body than those who are sedentary. This research also indicates that this size increase can occur after only six months of regular, moderate aerobic exercise.[24] Just think—you could become even *more* brilliant in six short months.

HOW EXERCISE AFFECTS THE WAY YOU MANAGE STRESS

Exercise increases your overall well-being, which puts more pep into your step. It accomplishes this by pumping up endorphins, which, you'll remember, are your brain's feel-good neurotransmitters. I like to call exercise "meditation in motion." This is how I feel when I exercise. It clears my mind and gives me a place to put all of the "stuff" rambling

---

23   Alan J. Gow, Mark E. Bastin, Susana Muñoz Maniega, Maria C. Valdés Hernández, Zoe Morris, Catherine Murray, Natalie A. Royle, John M. Starr, Ian J. Deary, and Joanna M. Wardlaw, "Neuroprotective Lifestyles and the Aging Brain: Activity, Atrophy, and White Matter Integrity," *Neurology* 79, no. 17 (2012), doi: 10.1212/WNL.0b013e3182703fd2.

24   Ibid.

around in my brain—making me constantly think and process. Exercise provides a way to release the tension that builds up in my brain and allows me to release my thoughts into the universe when I have no more room for ideas or learning.

I have not found anything else (not even meditation) that works quite as well to alleviate irritation and frustration from the day as much as working up a sweat. It simply works. As you begin to shed daily tensions through physical movement, you will also find that you can suddenly focus on a single task, while remaining more optimistic and clear minded than before. If you have trouble staying focused and your patience is gone, you can remedy this problem by adding regular daily body movement to your routine. It truly is that simple.

So, please tell me… if someone offered you a quick solution to better concentration and memory, less tension with clear focus, and a way to release your pent-up frustrations, all while making yourself look and feel great, why in the world would you not do it? You'd have to be half crazy not to. Just saying.

I *also* love the way that exercise builds self-confidence and courage in women. It helps women feel more comfortable in their own bodies, while improving how they look at themselves both physically and emotionally. It reduces depression, seasonal affective disorder, and mood swings. Most of all, exercise gives women a sense of command over their bodies and radically changes the way they manage day-to-day stress. Daily movement to the point of sweating helps women feel as if they have accomplished something, which for brilliant women is key.

HOW PHYSICAL ACTIVITY SUPPORTS THE STRESS GLAND FUNCTION

We're back to the adrenals… the glands dealing with the crux of the problem. Remember, adrenal fatigue is the layperson's term for hypothalamic-pituitary-adrenal (HPA) axis dysregulation, and this condition causes your body to stop responding to stress appropriately—which can include the stress of exercise. That's why it is important that you are aware that there is a downside to overdoing it with exercise coupled with excessive stress. With our on-the-go culture, where we work hard, play hard, and sometimes exercise too hard, we are not giving our bodies the needed downtime to recover. And many people with adrenal fatigue exercise too hard or begin exercising with too rigorous workouts for the condition they are in (not their physical condition but their stress/adrenal condition). They push themselves to the point of exhaustion and land on their face for three days wondering what happened to them.

The fact is, many women today are overexercising. (Don't get too excited by that news. I want to be careful even talking about this, because the number of women underexercising far outweighs the ones who are abusing exercise, but it is still important, and I need to touch on this.) Marathon runners, triathletes, or even women who want to start shedding fat—but are also overly stressed—need to be aware that too much high-intensity exercise can further deplete the adrenal glands, which will only make them feel worse. The key here is that you need to listen to your body. If you are feeling even more worn out and exhausted after exercise, you are depleting yourself with exercise, and you need to switch gears and readjust before you burn out.

Many overachieving women go from doing nothing to joining a fast-paced CrossFit class only to then wonder why they feel so weak after the workout or get hurt so easily. Other women who run races and keep pushing themselves to run longer distances sometimes find that it no longer makes them feel good, but they keep at it because they think it is good for them. Well, at one point in their lives it might have been, but when your adrenal function is compromised, it becomes a matter of simply not being able to muster up enough cortisol or adrenaline to get through the training. It is like running on fumes. It doesn't work, it is not good for you, and eventually you will break down.

Our bodies are similar to a car (only way more sophisticated, of course), and they need to run smoothly with perfect synchronization of numerous organs and systems or else the whole thing will start to deteriorate. With chronic stress and adrenal compromise, the body is drained and lacking energy, like a car running out of gas. Then, as the hormones are dysregulated, suddenly the body does not handle radical changes well—like going from sedentary to running a 5K in the same week (like how a car's faulty transmission makes it harder to switch gears).

The key to starting an exercise regimen when you feel exhausted and hung over from stress-induced adrenal fatigue is to first gain some control over your core functions (hormones, diet, and adrenal support strategies), which will put some "gas" into your body. Meanwhile, you can begin daily movement with something simple, like daily walks outside (nature is key for recovery). Exercise is a vital part of your stress recovery plan, and if done properly (slowly working up to more challenging routines), it will help boost your adrenal function instead of tanking your energy state further.

SITTING DOWN AND LOOKING AT A COMPUTER ALL DAY WILL EVENTUALLY KILL YOU!

Sorry for the scary language, but here's the truth you probably already knew but might need to be reminded of: Sit less, move more, live longer. There should be a sign posted on your computer. No matter how healthy you are, sitting for long periods of time is a risk factor for early death. There is now documented research showing a direct relationship between the time spent sitting and early death.[25] As the total sitting time increases, so does your risk for early death. The good news is that if you can manage

---

25   Mark D. Peterson, Aruna V. Sarma, and Paul M. Gordon, "Sitting Time and All-Cause Mortality Risk," *Archives of Internal Medicine* 172, no. 16 (2012), doi: 10.1001/archinternmed.2012.2527.

your routine and sit for less than 30 minutes at a time, you will have the lowest risk for early death. That is a pretty simple change that is definitely worth making.

So, for every 30 minutes you sit, you need to get up, move around, or walk for five minutes at a brisk pace. Even better, start using a stand-up desk with some exercise bands close by to work out your muscles in between emails. You'll both reduce health risks and clear your mind. It is vital that all brilliant women understand that as you age, your physical and mental function decline and you become more sedentary. So you have to try to reverse this by moving more while you are healthy and able. As we become more successful and more driven and pushed for more production in our professional lives, we sit more and forgo moving our body, thinking that makes us more productive. But this is the exact opposite of what we should be doing.

HOW TO EXERCISE AND EAT HEALTHY WHEN TIME IS LIMITED

It's easy to feel motivated to exercise after reading a blog about someone who's looking great after a four-week overhaul program, but it's another thing to actually put that program into practice. We are all busy people, and we rightfully think that we don't have the time to add one more thing. Yet when something really important comes up, we somehow find the time to do it or take care of it. The truth is that we don't put proper priority on exercise. So I'd like to propose that if you are truly too busy to exercise (or at least think you are), then you should consider combining exercise with other tasks, making it short and sweet and worth your while. The tips that follow will help you get started.

10 Tips for Organizing Your Time to Move Your Body

Here are 10 helpful tips for combining exercise into your daily routine that are guaranteed to keep you from going right over the edge.

1. Put your shoes on right when you get out of bed, when you have no distractions, and start early. This could mean getting up 30 minutes earlier. Before you say that's too early, here's the fix: Simply go to bed 30 minutes earlier. Easy, right?

2. At lunch, take a walk with a coworker and get some business dealt with at the same time.

3. Take your kids outside and move your body as fast as you can for 10–20 minutes. They'll love it!

4. Play ball with your kids instead of wasting a ridiculous amount of your precious time on social media.

5. Take exercise bands with you to work and use them in between emails. At home, have them out while watching TV, and spend the first ten minutes of your favorite show doing a band workout on four body parts while watching your show.

6. Call your grandmother or mother while you are on your exercise bike or out on a walk or a hike in nature.

7. Get a partner to work out with you. The most successful women I know need accountability (like me).

8. Listen to books on tape that teach you something new or expand your horizons while you exercise.

9. Meditate while you are working out (yes, this works) by playing a favorite app on your phone specifically designed for this. I love this. It sets my day exactly in line with my intentions.

10. Every time you go to the bathroom during the day, do ten lunges or squats followed by ten very slow wall push-ups (feet away from the wall, with hands on the wall slowly moving in to touch your chest on the wall). Don't worry about people watching you; they will join in after they realize how amazing you are looking.

The big trick to making sure that all these tips can help you is this: Schedule. Schedule. Schedule. You need to keep exercise in your schedule as a no-cancellation appointment. Make a commitment to be committed to this, so that not only can you shed body fat but your mood, sleep, and ability to manage stress will all be optimized. See the door of exercise, kick it down, and walk through it like a boss.

Quick Cardio Fat Burning

The long workouts of the past are now being replaced with quick-cardio, fat-burning, high-intensity plans that will save you time while helping you achieve real results. Here are seven suggestions for a metabolism-boosting, muscle-building workout routine that will not cramp your schedule or put you over the edge. Get ready to sweat.

1. Beginners should start with ten minutes per day in the morning and evening. Those more used to exercise should start with 15–20 minutes. Begin with a one-minute warm-up: Walk at a moderate pace, taking longer strides and stretching out your calves and hamstrings. Then, start to move at a pace that you feel is nearly as fast as you can go. You can slow down for 30 seconds to one minute if you need to catch your breath. Then, repeat until the time is up. If you want to switch it up, do anything that raises your heart rate: walk, jump rope, treadmill, dance in your home to music—anything. How easy is that?

2. Increase this workout time by five minutes each week until you can sustain 20 minutes with one- to two-minute recovery periods every five minutes, moving as fast as you can while walking, jumping, dancing, or whatever you choose.

3. Stay consistent with your workout times as much as possible so that you are better able to regulate your blood sugar. This is also why you should always do morning cardio on an empty stomach. And consider taking a quick walk outside before you leave the office at the end of the day, which would also normally be on an empty stomach. Doing this will help you burn up to 200 percent more calories.

4. To combine activities, take a coworker or your child with you in a stroller and move your body while talking, which increases your heart rate. Listen to motivational or educational books on tape, and learn as you go. Or use the recorder on your phone to collect thoughts about what you need to do the rest of the day or to meditate while walking. Walking meditation and setting intentions while you work out will completely change your attitude and the course of your day for the better.

5. Make the timing of your workout a priority so it does not get bumped for something else. Use the ten tips in the previous list. Start your day by getting out of bed and putting your shoes on. Get up 30 minutes earlier if you need to.

6. When you feel overly stressed, don't reach for a muffin or a donut, which will make you feel awful. Instead, put your workout shoes on and leave the work place for a ten-minute, fast-paced walk. Get some endorphins going, and you will mentally and emotionally process the rest of the day better.

7. One alternative, which is called metabolic training, takes less time and is more effective than an hour of brisk walking as far as caloric burning and exercise performance are concerned. This is achieved by doing eight rounds of 30-second intervals of high-intensity movements that get your heart rate up. With this training, you walk, run, jog, cycle, dance, or doing anything as fast and as hard as you can for 20 seconds to get your heart rate up, followed by ten seconds of resting. Then, you repeat this interval eight times consecutively over four minutes. Flat-out effort is required to do this type of exercising correctly. If you finish the series with ease, you are not working hard enough, but if your last few sets are feeling a bit impossible, you're doing it right.

If you have done these metabolic training exercises for four minutes over a period of one to two months, it may be time to increase the timing and push for 15–20 minutes, as your body will likely have gotten used to the old routine. Also, switch up the types of cardio you are doing and rotate between them in your workouts. (For instance, cycling and walking could easily be rotated within the same workout.)

Also, remember when recovering from adrenal stress issues, do not exceed 20 minutes of training a day, and get an extra half hour of sleep at night for added metabolism boosting. Yes, you do build muscle and even make human growth hormone while you sleep, which will give you an added boost for the weight loss you are looking for.

Quick Strength Training Metabolism Boosters

I am a big fan of cramming as much as possible into every available second of the day, especially for things I don't usually think I have time for. (It's a little manic, I know.) Lifting, weight resistance, and body building are a few things I would neglect if I didn't have creative ways of fitting them into my day. I love exercise bands, exercise balls, and using my body weight for lifting and building muscle. I personally *never* go to the gym. Some people thrive there, but it's not for me. I love the outdoors far better. In nature, I can clear my head and heal. It's important that you find what works for you, as long as you are getting exercise and building muscle.

Building muscle is paramount to your fitness journey. Lean muscle increases your metabolism, has more than twice the blood flow of fat, and stores no toxins (as fat does). It makes your arms, legs, and butt look smooth and firm (good-bye cellulite). Most importantly, muscle provides a strong foundation for bones and joints, improves posture, and reduces stress on the body, which helps prevent injuries. And, obviously, strong arms and legs will give you confidence—and they're nice to look at.

When using weight resistance to build muscles, exercises should be intense enough for your muscles to be working and becoming slightly fatigued, but not so much that you get shaky, weak, or excessively sore. If you are lifting weights or using your own body weight to exercise (sit-ups, push-ups, lunges), you should perform several sets of ten or more. With each set, you should do as many as it takes to get to the point where you are fatigued in the muscle group you are working. You should become increasingly fatigued with each set, but not to the point where you cannot complete the set. And remember, exercise doesn't have to happen at the gym. You can work out in the comfort of your own home, in your office, or in a hotel room, if you travel for work often.

There are many types of home or gym training aids that will work your muscles. The easiest to start with is exercise bands. They usually come with full-body workout descriptions and pictures included for all levels of fitness, and they are easy to take anywhere. Try to have your exercise bands or other exercise tools at home and work or anywhere else you are spending time so they are easy to grab. The following are some easy ways you can strength train and boost your metabolism:

1. Set your phone alarm for your workouts during the day. You can do your strength and cardio separately or put them together. For strength training, your goal is to work four body parts each day. This will take you less than 12 minutes and can be done right after your quick-cardio workout, later in the morning, in the evening, or even by taking short breaks at work.

2. Superset each body part. Which, for example, means do one set (of 10–20 reps) of biceps, then one set of shoulders, then one set of upper back, and then one set of triceps. Then, repeat two more sets of each, with 30-second breaks between the three sets.

3. Rotate body parts daily, if you can, so you are focusing on a different set of four each day.

4. You can also use your own body weight to exercise, such as when doing sit-ups, push-ups, lunges, and squats.

You won't believe how fast this simple plan can reshape your body (especially if you are working on your diet at the same time). Muscle training will improve the way your skin looks and how you feel about your body. It will give you a better margin for error with your eating, create more confidence, and power up your sex drive. It is a big metabolism booster, which enables your body to burn fat for up to 48 hours after the workout has finished. Now *that* is worth it.

Yoga for Flexibility and Stress Control

Consider adding one to two short yoga sessions per week to promote strength, flexibility, and a deeper mind-body connection. This will improve your body's reaction to stress and teach you how to harness your mind against it. Better yet, yoga will help you age better by promoting longer, leaner, more flexible muscles. It is clearing and centering, and it improves longevity. Here are some easy ways to start:

1. Find a good yoga app on your phone that is specifically for stress, and follow along once a week. Get a mat and practice yoga for 30 minutes at work (if you can) or at home.

2. Consider using a roller ball on your muscles to keep your connective tissue from getting sticky, which can cause pain and stiff joints. This should be done ten minutes daily. This is also a wonderful way to reduce cellulite. And it feels great too.

Organize, Prep, and Go

I think we can all agree that preparation leads to success, and to be a successful woman, preparation is key. While exercise and moving your body are imperative for stress control and slowing the aging process, every expert says the same thing about fat loss: It's 80 percent diet. Let's face it, if you are trying to lose body fat and look better, but your diet is in shambles, you can exercise your brains out and still not lose weight. So, taking the time to prepare your food and schedule your exercise will be the key to your success in looking good and feeling great. Not prepping ahead of time will likely leave you running for chocolate instead of broccoli when crunch time comes.

My goal is to help you treat your exercise time as you would your business or career: You want to get the best bang for your buck. Your training sessions will be far more effective if you are eating the right foods for promoting your muscles and discouraging fat storage. The best way to be successful at this is by preparing the right food ahead of time. No matter what particular diet you are on—keto, Paleo, low carb, balanced carbs, Mediterranean, or intermittent fasting—you need to give yourself adequate prep time.

The tips for prepping that follow will help you save time and money while making the most of your workouts. Try to spend one afternoon a week prepping for the week ahead. I find Sunday afternoon works best for me, but any day is fine.

1. Plan out what you need for dinner each night. Prepare your menu for the week with a quick shopping list and head to the grocery store.

2. You can also prep a Crock-Pot full of chicken, cook up some quinoa, oatmeal, boiled eggs, and clean and chop veggies. Put them into individual servings. Take bags of prepared organic lettuce and put them into separate bowls with lids as ready-made salads. Or consider glass jars for layered premade salads. You can even turn on some music and get your family to join in to help with prep time. A little creativity can make anything fun.

3. Fill two to three bottles with lemon water to take to work with you.

4. Cut up chicken, turkey, veggies, and lettuce leaves to act as your bread for sandwiches, and get lunch bags ready and ice packs in the freezer.

5. Get your workout clothes ready, and text your workout partner to meet you at specific times each day.

6. Get to bed early by getting ready for the next day early. Insist that your family help you so you can get to bed on time.

7. Remove the junk food from your house. Your family doesn't need it either.

8. Make sure you have enough groceries to get you through the week.

9. Try to cook more dinner than you need so you have lunch for you

and your family the next day. Leftover salmon or chicken or meat on top of salads the next day is perfect—and it will save you time.

10. Spend your lunch break walking instead of going out to lunch. This is fun and often much more enjoyable. Keep walking shoes and exercise bands at work and home.

Time Wasters to Avoid

While I think some women are naturals at capitalizing on every second of the day and maximizing their time, others struggle with getting caught up in the day-to-day minutia that leaves them feeling strapped and unable to fit in all the things they want to do. The key here is to eliminate whatever it is you are doing that is not explicitly helping you take care of yourself.

I have always encouraged my patients who are experiencing toxic stress in their lives to examine how they are spending their time so they can begin the tedious task of scheduling every minute of their waking hours. I understand that this sounds somewhat militant, but it can help you take the first steps in eliminating toxic stress in your life, and it will be glaringly obvious where your time is being wasted when you do this.

Nowadays, scheduling your day is even easier because of all the wonderful apps available to help you schedule your time. I would suggest, if you have an inkling that you are a bit of time waster, that you invest in a handheld physical planner or an app that helps you plan your day so you will see exactly what you are doing with your time. To continue to be brilliant, we need to harness our time and make the most of it; that's the only way we will have enough of it to take care of ourselves and our families. This ultimately boils down to priorities. Number one is you and your health, number two is your family, and number three is your brilliant career and the gifts you have to give to others.

So let's take a look at the stats on time wasting:

- The average person spends three hours per day on social media. Social media has nothing to do with their career or their health, so that is a big waste of time.

- Women can spend at least two hours per day surfing the internet—and let's be honest, that has nothing to do with self-improvement, business development, career advancement, or anything that could potentially make our lives better or happier. We are often spending more money than we should by surfing the internet and engaging in impulse online shopping at night as a pastime.

- The average person listens to one or more hours of news each day, which fills you with fear, is depressing, and makes you feel as if you have no control, while biasing you that the world is an awful place to live. No, thank you.

- On average, we spend two hours a day focusing, worrying, and talking about hypothetical situations that are not even part of our reality. We let our brains wander and make up situations and perceptions about our lives, jobs, friends, and family that are based on our own emotions rather than reality. This is useless and, honestly, a little insane. So stop worrying. Live your life and harness your power to control your brain and your thoughts.

- We are guilty of too much multitasking. Interruptions can waste hours of time each day, because they prevent you from focusing on the project right in front of you. So if you are answering emails, you should not be answering texts at the same time. While you may think your brain is capable of multitasking, *it is not*. And if you continue to do it, you will pay the price by forgetting, losing your focus, and wasting your beautiful brain. Tune in and focus on one thing at a time. Let your mind seize each moment for itself.

- Women can waste an absolutely staggering amount of time each day looking for their keys, phone, computer cords, pens, documents on their computer, or whatever else they need because they either haven't created a dedicated space for these things or set them down somewhere while they were distracted by other things. These situations send up your stress alarms big time.

Ladies, here's your takeaway from these frankly depressing statistics: Harness your time and get things under control. Your health and happiness are your number-one priority. Stop wasting your precious time with too many excuses, and use it to get your body moving, feeding yourself endorphins that will help your brilliance shine.

Your Morning Ritual

Consider incorporating a morning ritual. To get started with this, go to bed—and then get up in the morning—one hour earlier than usual. Each morning, make the following priorities: meditation for ten minutes, exercising your body for 30 minutes, and spending 10 minutes preparing your food for the day (lunch, snacks, water bottles, and getting food out on the counter for dinner or throwing it all in a Crock-Pot to start cooking while you are working). Try to always take lunch, snacks, and water with you to work if you can. If you work from home or are a stay-at-home mom, get your daily plan organized early in the morning before everyone wakes up and starts trying to "help." This quiet time in the morning is sacred, and you need to take advantage of it when your head is clear and no one is calling, texting, or emailing you.

The only way you can or will accomplish this is to get to bed earlier. I cannot emphasize how vital this is for your long-term survival and recovery. I know this might not be possible every night, but most nights it will be. Your brain is better in the morning when you have refueled in this way. And you'll be better able to move through your daily tasks if you have slept well.

FAST-TRACK PLAN FOR EXERCISE TO RESHAPE AND REBUILD

Moving your body will save you. It will make you a better, happier person and will improve how you age. No matter how busy you are, please exercise. Get outside, experience nature, cleanse your spirit and mind, and know that this will allow you to be even more brilliant. For those of you looking to jump-start a healthy lifestyle, try following this simple fast-track plan.

- Plan out the food you need for your meals each week.

- Find a workout partner or someone to keep you accountable for exercise. Consider getting a trainer to come to your home and give you a workout using bands, kettlebells, or your own body weight. Then, have the trainer come back and make a new plan for you every four weeks to measure your success, change things up, and test your body fat. Paying someone is good motivation to get your money's worth, and accountability is key. Remember, the most successful women need someone to keep them accountable, because they are too busy taking care of everything and everyone else.

- Make a weekly grocery list. Keep the list on your counter and jot down items during the week. Consider sending someone to do your grocery shopping for you, which is a major time saver.

- Stop eating junk when you are stressed and have low blood sugar. Instead, prepare for the worst and do not let yourself get desperate. Get protein bars, nuts, seeds, and healthy snacks to stash at your desk and in your car, and don't let yourself make poor choices.

- You *must* move your body daily. I don't even care if it is a quick ten-minute power walk between meetings. Keep workout shoes in your car and at work. Simply put them on and go. Your nervous system will thank you.

- Try not to sit for more than 30 minutes at a time. The easiest way to do this is to switch to a stand-up desk. You should also start getting up to move around and stretch in meetings. No one will mind if you do it respectfully, and it will keep you feeling more energetic while burning calories.

- Document your weight weekly, and chart monthly measurements of your waist, hips, bust, arms, and thighs.

- Each week, write down your fitness goals and ask yourself, "What have I done to improve my physical health, and how does this make me feel emotionally and mentally?" This will help you stay on track.

- Consider using a fitness app or an exercise watch to chart your progress. Get into a fitness group challenge using a favorite app, and work hard to compete with others so you are having some fun killing your competition. Get in 8,000–10,000 steps per day. Move. Move. Move. Whatever exercise you choose, commit to establishing it as a habit. It will take six weeks to lock it in.

- Join a class at your club, and have a friend meet you there. This can be a fun way to stay accountable.

- Walk before you run. Build up your fitness level gradually, and don't go crazy and kill yourself or strain your muscles by trying to overdo it. This is a long-term plan.

- Understand you may be the type of person who hates any type of exercise for as long as you are breathing. That's okay. However, you still *have* to exercise, and it's imperative to commit—no excuses. You will live longer, be happier, and be more successful. Period.

- Take one day off per week and do something fun, such as going for a hike in the mountains, taking a horseback ride, going to the river, or just doing something to unwind while still relaxing and unplugging.

- Breathe. You will severely delay your recovery if you don't start taking some deep breaths. Taking as few as five deep breaths can switch your nervous system from a sympathetic ("keyed up") to a parasympathetic ("rest and digest") mode, which will keep you from having a total meltdown before the day even begins.

Fitness Success Story

In late 2015, a very lean, overachieving triathlete named Jordyn came to my office. She was an executive who was killing it in her job and traveling from city to city for work. She had been a runner most of her life, and at the age of 48, she was still winning triathlons and was addicted to running. Jordyn was goal oriented and tried to fit in two hours of exercise each day.

She did get the most out of her time—she ran with headphones on and would listen to business books on tape as she rode her bike. She was competing in races three to four times yearly while working 50–60 hours every week. One of her goals was to compete in a national competition, and she felt she could place in it if she kicked up her training. But, unfortunately, her body was starting to fail. She had intense fatigue and pain and suffered from injuries she had not had in the past. Overall, she was feeling lousy.

She knew something was wrong, and it was. She had overdone it. Her body was trying to send her the message that there was simply no fuel left in her tank. The adrenaline that had kept her juggling everything had finally run out, and she was running on fumes. We did some lab work and discovered her testosterone, DHEA, thyroid, and estradiol levels were low. Her body fat was 5 percent, which you might think means she was extremely healthy, but on paper, her labs looked like she was an 80-year-old woman. I had no other option but to advise her to readjust her goals and to stop pushing herself excessively with competition. This was the only way she could give her body the rest it needed so it could recover.

She fought me on this for a year, but eventually she got so sick she had to listen. I gave her a relatively simple treatment plan to get her back to her optimal health.

HER GAME PLAN INCLUDED THE FOLLOWING:

- Immediately fixing all of her hormone levels with bioidentical hormones

- Stopping her running workouts completely until her health stabilized

- Starting a more low-impact workout routine with casual bike rides, shorter sessions of swimming, and group spin classes

- Eating more healthy fats and protein to help get her to a healthier weight

This plan literally saved her life. Today she has gained 20 pounds (very much needed), her hormones are vibrant, her skin looks amazing, she lifts weights to help build muscle, and she now coaches other athletic women on how to refuel *before* burnout. She has also become an amazing advocate for women who can't seem to make movement part of their life but so desperately want to look and feel good. She is a superwoman coach and intimately knows firsthand how you can hurt your body with excessive exercise combined with excessive stress.

(8)

The Brilliance of Sex: The Easiest (and Most Fun) Way to Look Younger, Feel Great, and Age Better

"Sex is part of nature. I go along with nature."
—*MARILYN MONROE*

A healthy sex drive is paramount to looking younger and feeling great. Take the quiz below to see where you fall on the sex drive spectrum.

QUIZ: DO YOU HAVE A HEALTHY SEX DRIVE?

1. Has your libido (sex drive) decreased in the past year? Y/N
2. Do you avoid intimate situations that may lead to sex? Y/N
3. Has your frequency of sex declined in the last several months or years? Y/N

4. Have you said "I'm just fine without sex" to yourself lately? Y/N

5. Do you have PMS, menopause, or premenopausal symptoms? Y/N

6. Have you noticed a loss of muscle strength with exercise? Y/N

7. Are you irritable or grumpy, or are you having trouble tolerating stress? Y/N

8. Do you argue with your partner about the frequency of sex you have? Y/N

9. Does your partner like to have sex more often than you? Y/N

10. Do you frequently feel exhausted for no reason? Y/N

11. Do you have trouble getting to sleep or staying asleep? Y/N

12. Do you feel overwhelmed and underappreciated? Y/N

13. Is your concentration or memory poor? Y/N

14. Does being touched sometimes make your skin crawl? Y/N

15. Do you have pain with sex? Y/N

16. Do you rarely think about sex? Y/N

17. Are you unhappy with your partner? Y/N

18. Is it more difficult to reach an orgasm than it once was? Y/N

19. Have you been diagnosed with high blood pressure, diabetes, or hypo-thyroidism? Y/N

20. Would you like to improve your sex life? Y/N

Total your number of yes answers and see the corresponding results:

1–6: You may have the beginning of female sexual decline. Keep reading to learn the signs and treatments to make sure you don't start losing out on sex.

7–12: "It's been *how* long?" You are most likely experiencing a combination of lifestyle disturbances and stress, leading to low sexual drive, and may be seeing signs of female sexual dysfunction with lowering or fluctuating levels of hormones.

13–20: Girl, you need more than to get laid! You may have an arousal disorder (sexual drive disorder) and are most likely experiencing toxic stress, relationship issues, orgasm disorder, and declining sexual hormone levels.

....

In case you scored a bit higher than you would like and are feeling a little overwhelmed, sad, guilty, or discouraged, don't give up. Keep reading. The information that follows will help you get started on your brilliantly awesome sex plan in no time. Trust me, you will be glad you did, as there truly is more in sex for you than you think—you just have to work for it.

WHY SEX HELPS WITH STRESS

Most of us know that healthy sex feels good and improves our relationships while giving us a bit of pep in our step the following day. However, most women have no idea that good sex releases hormones that improve how our entire body works.

Stress is a major cause of a lousy sex drive. Excessive stress puts strain on our adrenals, making us feel exhausted and not interested in adding one more thing to the never-ending daily list of things to do. (And sex does feel like a task when you're stressed.) This unfair, vicious cycle of high stress, fatigue, and infrequent sex robs us of cashing in on all of the proven stress-busting benefits of good sex.

Orgasms are one of the best stress relievers available to women, as they help us on an emotional, mental, and physical level. But the crazy (though probably unsurprising) thing is that the most common reason a woman cannot orgasm is *stress*, which only perpetuates the cycle.

The adrenal glands secrete hormones that pump up your libido. But when your stress glands become run down from daily demands, causing physical and mental exhaustion, the last thing any woman wants is to jump into bed with her partner for more performance-based work, especially if orgasms are not easily achieved.

Women dealing with high stress are in survival mode and are simply worried about getting through their day, not procreating (and certainly not pleasuring). Ultimately, this robs us of the very benefits we need to sustain ourselves in the midst of high stress. Crazy, isn't it?

For many women, having sex is just one more thing they don't have time for, aren't into, or are simply too exhausted to even think about. But what if I told you sex could reduce your stress, enhance your level of happiness, help you age better, and control your weight? What if you were convinced that you could get as much if not more than your partner out of sex? Jackpot, right? Well, it's true.

As more research is churned out on the health benefits of sex, it's becoming clear that having a healthy sex life is essential to achieving a long, balanced life. Sex as a health treatment was recommended in the 1930s, when doctors prescribed orgasm as a treatment for women with hysteria who could not adjust socially. And, sure, the very definition of *hysteria* is pretty sexist (with male physicians prescribing sex for hysterical women…), but the point is that even then they somehow knew sex was a slam dunk for treating psychological or mental stress.

Today, sex studies for women and men continue to show that this amazing gift we have built right into our bodies can release hormones that help regulate stress. University of Michigan researchers demonstrated that orgasms increase estrogen and help women release oxytocin (the love hormone), which lowers and helps stabilize the stress hormones.[26] Oxytocin is a pretty incredible hormone; it makes us happy, creates bonds between people, lowers our body pain, relieves depression, staves off anxiety, and helps balance other hormones that work synergistically to keep us at our best.

Stress increases the release of ACTH (adrenocorticotropic hormone), a stress hormone signal from the brain, but with satisfying orgasms, the hormone oxytocin is released, which provides a sense of calmness and

---

26   Sari M. Van Anders, Lori Brotto, Janine Farrell, and Morag Yule, "Associations Among Physiological and Subjective Sexual Response, Sexual Desire, and Salivary Steroid Hormones in Healthy Premenopausal Women," *The Journal of Sexual Medicine* 6, no. 3 (2009): 739–751, doi: 10.1111/j.1743-6109.2008.01123.x.

relaxation to counteract the effects of ACTH. Orgasms also increase the brain chemical dopamine, which provides a sense of well-being, even in the midst of high stress. Overall, orgasms immediately induce a calming effect on the nervous system and move us from a state of "survival" to a state of "rest and relax," which our entire system is crying out for at the end of a stressful day.

With high stress, there is something known as the *pregnenolone steal*, which further compromises a woman's balanced state. The pregnenolone steal occurs when, under high stress, the hormone pregnenolone (which is highest on the hormone manufacturing chain) makes a switch to producing more stress hormones like cortisol to manage all of your daily stress and, in turn, siphons energy away from making other hormones, like estradiol, progesterone, and testosterone that keep your sex drive optimal. I find all of this particularly interesting because the more stressed women are, the less sex they have. Likewise, the more stressed they become, the more hormones are diverted away from fixing that, creating a compromised sex drive and sexual functioning. This is yet another bad cycle that we find ourselves in with stress that not only tips us out of balance but also adversely affects our relationships with those we love the most.

One of the best ways our bodies can cope with stress is through sleep, and it turns out that having sex before bed can help with that. Sex-induced oxytocin promotes deeper, more restorative sleep, and vasopressin, another chemical associated with good sleep and inducing sleepiness, is also released during orgasm. Sleep is one of the most important ingredients for helping brilliant women recover, so if you are struggling to get to sleep, remember that having an orgasm would be a much better choice than popping another sleeping pill. A powerful orgasm is thought to be equivalent to two to three milligrams of Valium. So, if good sex promotes relaxation, restorative sleep, and optimal mood (not to mention the satisfaction of a blow-your-mind orgasm) that results in ultimately being more balanced and productive, why would we not partake regularly?

To appreciate another way sex helps us beat stress, we have to talk about the circuit system in the brain of all women that is involved in feelings of happiness, called the limbic system. This system is deep in the brain, and it's more active when we are rewarded (not stressed). Unsurprisingly, this system is easily activated with sex (and anything else that we enjoy). During sex, more blood flows to the brain, and more neurons fire with noted high levels of brain activity. Much of this deep brain circuit also runs on the hormone dopamine, and when we partake in pleasurable, enjoyable activities (like good sex), it causes the brain cells to release more dopamine, which drives the firing of the brain to occur faster. So, sex may not only make us happier, but it might also make us smarter! And for stressed-out women today, we need to engage in pleasurable activities like sex that naturally raise dopamine to keep us from habituating on other things that are not healthy for us (like food, alcohol, and drugs).

HEALTHY HORMONES RELEASED WITH GOOD SEX

It is fairly well known that the act of sex sets off a cascade of hormones that trigger pleasure, happiness, and bonding. And while we have already covered the fact that women need testosterone to help promote a healthy sexual drive, it can also work the other way around. New research has shown that testosterone is released in women during sexy thoughts, kissing, cuddling, foreplay, and orgasm. And since testosterone increases the sex drive (the more you have it, the more you want it), this makes you more confident and brave—and ultimately more likely to take sex to completion. All this is to say that sexual function and drive are a lot like a muscle. If we don't use it, we will lose it.

When testosterone is at an optimal level in women (and remember, sometimes women need to have testosterone optimized through testing and treatment), it will add to the fire of sexual desire and give you more confidence, while also improving the efficiency of orgasm. Additionally, on the other side of the hormone spectrum, sex also promotes healthy estrogen levels that keep vaginal tissues elastic, lubricated, and youthful.

The love hormone, oxytocin, is also released during an orgasm (and can be prescribed if someone is chronically low in it). This hormone is needed to regulate other hormone levels impaired by stress and the menstrual cycle. With oxytocin deficiency, women experience more weight gain, emotional distress, impaired cognitive function, and even increases in cancer rates. Some sexual health experts believe that the clitoris is a reset button for oxytocin. By having a clitoral orgasm, oxytocin is released, which improves multiple aspects of our physical and emotional well-being.

SEX IMPROVES YOUR OVERALL HEALTH

Let me stop beating around the bush here and simply say outright what you were probably all hoping to hear. Several studies now show that sex is not just good, but *great* for our health. It can protect against heart disease and osteoporosis, stave off dementia, and even improve your mood. There are so many benefits to the release of oxytocin (which I like to call the cuddling hormone) for brilliant women today. Oxytocin reduces the symptoms of irritable bowel syndrome or nervous stomach, improves digestion, and helps cure constipation and gastrointestinal inflammation. Additionally, it helps lower blood pressure and provides a sense of calmness and peacefulness to our entire nervous system.

For any younger women out there still building their families, here's something else you should know: Good sex even improves fertility by increasing contractions of the uterus, helping to "suck in" the semen released during male orgasm. So don't come at it as though you're accomplishing a task; enjoy it!

Sex also protects women from incontinence, as it is a good workout for the pelvic floor muscles. The muscles that are involved with urination need regular exercise, and sex does just that, improving blood flow, strength, and circulation to the entire pelvic floor, which reduces the chances of urine leaking and uterine prolapse later in life. After having children and with our busy lives, the Kegel exercises (to strengthen the muscles in the pelvic floor) are often lost in the shuffle, but having regular sex is a great substitute, as it can provide a much-needed exercise for the pelvic floor muscles.

Sex Can Help You Live Longer

Just when you thought there were no antiaging longevity supplements or skin care products left to try, who would have thought that a good roll in the hay could help you live longer. Well, I'm here to share that orgasms can in fact add *years* to your life. Women who have regular (twice weekly) orgasms have been shown to live longer than those who do not.[27] Researchers point out that it's more than just the orgasm that's good for women, and chalk this extended lifespan up to women being happier and having a healthier relationship with their significant other as well.[28] Think about this for a minute: You can live longer by simply having a mind-blowing orgasm at least twice weekly. This is a win-win, ladies!

Sex can even have a protective effect on the heart. A study at Queen's University in Belfast found that having sex three times a week could cut

27 Carl D. Reimers, Guido Knapp, and Anne Kerstin Reimers, "Does Physical Activity Increase Life Expectancy? A Review of the Literature," *Journal of Aging Research* 11 (2012): 243958, doi:10.1155/2012/243958.

28 Carl J. Charnetski and Francis X. Brennan, "Sexual Frequency and Salivary Immunoglobulin A (IgA)," *Psychological Reports* 94, no. 3 (2004): 839–844, doi:10.2466/pr0.94.3.839-844.

the risk of a heart attack or stroke in half.[29] And another study in Israel found that women who had two orgasms a week were up to 30 percent less likely to have heart disease than those who didn't enjoy sex or didn't orgasm.[30] One reason for this could be that women who have regular sex are typically less depressed, which decreases their chances of getting heart disease.

Orgasms are also good for the immune system. DHEA (another hormone released when you climax) helps to keep your immune system running more efficiently. Sex also provides an overall lymphatic massage (when you're doing it right, at least, *wink*), improving your body's natural detoxification process, which helps keep you from getting sick in the first place. On top of all this, it also improves digestion. And improved digestion, as we've discussed, boosts the immune system and even prevents cancer.

Studies have shown that women who have sex a few times per week have much higher amounts of the antibody immunoglobulin A (IgA) than those who have sex less than once a week.[31] What does that mean? Well, IgA is the first line of defense against colds and flu, among a host of other illnesses. Sex is good for you in so many ways.

I don't know about you, but I sleep like a baby after a satisfying orgasm. Turns out, this is yet another health benefit of sex. The deep, restorative sleep following sex has been shown in numerous studies to extend your lifespan. Sex is also good for your bones, because the oxytocin released during orgasm increases the density of bones and helps to prevent bone loss associated with aging and osteoporosis.

29 George Davey Smith, Stephen Frankel, and John Yarnell, "Sex and Death: Are They Related? Findings from the Caerphilly Cohort Study," *BMJ* 315 (1997): 1641, doi: 10.1136/bmj.315.7123.1641.

30 Steven M. Butler and David A. Snowdon, "Trends in Mortality in Older Women: Findings from the Nun Study," *Journal of Gerontology: Social Sciences* 51B, no. 4 (1996): S201–S208, https://www.ncbi.nlm.nih.gov/pubmed/8673649.

31 Carl J. Charnetski and Francis X. Brennan, "Sexual Frequency and Salivary Immunoglobulin A (IgA)," *Psychological Reports* 94, no. 3 (2004): 839–844, doi:10.2466/pr0.94.3.839-844.

Sex Is Good for Your Brain

Sex can even sharpen a women's mind and enhance focus, memory, and concentration. Evidence has emerged showing that older people who are sexually active are less likely to have dementia. This is because the more sex you have, amazingly, the more cells you can grow in your brain. Sex also increases blood flow to the brain, which in turn increases the oxygen supply to the brain, making it easier to think clearly. MRI scans of the brain have shown that during orgasm, the neurons in the brain are more active and use more oxygen. This increased demand for oxygen-rich blood then facilitates the delivery of a fresh supply of nutrients to the brain to keep it healthy longer.

Sex Is the Cure for What Ails You

Finally, orgasms are also fantastic at reducing body pain. With many of my patients, I have witnessed the damaging effects of chronic pain. These women age right before my eyes. Chronic body pain upsets the entire stress system, and having good sex can help combat this. Orgasms block pain signals and inhibit their transmission from the spinal cord to the brain even long after the orgasm is over, so the perception of pain is ultimately reduced. Because of this effect, studies have also shown that the pain threshold is higher in women who have regular sex, which has been found to be equivalent to the effect of morphine.[32] A study was performed and published in *Experimental Biology and Medicine* that showed when the participants inhaled oxytocin and then had their fingers pricked, their pain threshold was lowered by half.[33] So maybe instead of turning a cold

---

32   Adam S. Sprouse-Blum, Greg Smith, Daniel Sugai, and Fereydoun Don Parsa, "Understanding Endorphins and Their Importance in Pain Management," *Hawaii Medical Journal* 69, no.3 (2010): 70–71, https://www.ncbi.nlm.nih.gov/pmc/articles/PMC3104618/.

33   Yu V. Uryvaev and G. A. Petrov, "Extremely Low Doses of Oxytocin Reduce Pain Sensitivity in Men," *Bulletin of Experimental Biology and Medicine* 122, no. 5 (1996): 1071–1073, doi: 10.1007/BF02447648.

shoulder to sex the next time you have a headache, think again... it could be just what the doctor ordered.

GOOD SEX REDUCES CRAVINGS, APPETITE, AND BELLY FAT

At its most basic level, sex increases blood flow and gets your heart pumping. Simply put, sex is a form of exercise and—at a caloric burn of 150–350 calories per session—it's a lot more fun than running laps. Have you ever noticed that women in new relationships often lose weight or how women come back after a relaxing getaway with their partner looking so amazing? Well, now you know why. The secret is that frequent sex creates the perfect vortex of appetite reduction, craving control, and enhanced mood. The release of oxytocin may also shift our motivational behavior from a desire to eat toward a desire to have more sex. Oxytocin also counteracts anxiety and depression by activating the brain chemicals that control how we eat (i.e., stress eating). Additionally, sex helps control the highs and lows of cortisol, which is well known for its role in boosting belly fat and increasing carbohydrate cravings. Overall, it seems that increasing the amount of sex you have can give you a better body, improved mood, more self-confidence, vibrancy, and an increased *desire* for more sex.

SEX BOOSTS SELF-ESTEEM, CONFIDENCE, AND IMPROVES RELATIONSHIPS

When you climax, your body releases chemicals called endorphins that make you feel great. An orgasm is basically nature's antidepressant (and without all the weird side effects). Other hormones are also released when you climax that can help improve your overall outlook on life and make you a happier person.

As I've mentioned, the hormone oxytocin is one of these hormones. It is linked to passion, intuition, and bonding. It improves relationships, increases a woman's and a man's sense of empathy, and lowers the guards between lovers while helping to increase a sense of trust and connection between them. It helps women feel more social (which is often lost during high stress) and enhances connections among coworkers. Higher levels of oxytocin relieve depression, create a sense of happiness, knock down negativity, and even help to eliminate postpartum depression. Oxytocin is also believed to improve the relationships between parents and children.

The psychological benefits of a healthy sex life are many. The feeling of extreme joy or elation you get after good sex lasts longer than you think. People who are sexually active are also less likely to have alexithymia. This is a personality trait characterized by the inability to express or understand emotions. Last, and of pretty great importance for most of us, sex helps you look younger—studies show making love three times a week in a stress-free relationship can make you look ten years younger, which for sure helps your self-esteem.

EIGHT SIGNS OF A BAD SEX LIFE

Bottom line: Busy women like us need support from our loved ones. We need to be nourished outside of our daily grind, and that includes sexually. Having a partner who takes more than they give is not only unhealthy, but it's also the last thing you need with an overcommitted life. I realize you may know all of this already. God knows analyzing relationships is about the only thing magazines cover these days, but I still want to skim over it in case you recognize yourself in any of these scenarios. If you do,

I recommend using this list as a way to recognize possible pitfalls of a bad sex life so you can then begin addressing them one by one.

1. Your partner has an orgasm every time, and you rarely or never have one. Are one or both of you under the impression that sex is all about their orgasm and not yours? Remember all of the things I have already shared with you on the benefits of good, healthy sex. You need to get your fair share of the benefit.

2. Your partner informs you that if you can't orgasm in five to ten minutes, there must be something wrong with you (the average female takes 20–30 minutes to achieve an orgasm, and that time may increase as you age). The good stuff takes time.

3. Sex ends when your partner has an orgasm. Don't accept this. Sex should end when both parties are satisfied.

4. Your partner doesn't realize that sex starts in the kitchen with communication and help. There should be some communication like, "How was your day" or "How are you doing?" Plus, your partner should help you in the evening so you are not run ragged by the time you are finally able to make your way to bed.

5. If your partner is a man, he is too rough during sex and has no idea where your clitoris is or how to manage it. The clitoris is highly sensitive and has thousands of nerve endings that cannot be overridden. Rough management of the clitoris can even reduce the overall sensation and create a numbing effect. Very light touching and intermittent changes in the amount of touch have shown to significantly increase a woman's sexual sensation and orgasm potential.

6. Kissing and cuddling is not part of the sexual encounter before or after. Women still need romance, and this is a huge turn-on for

women that people (men especially) often forget about or simply never do. Kissing is also important because it kick-starts multiple mechanisms in the brain, releasing chemicals that lower stress and help a woman relax.

7. Your partner keeps asking you to do sexual favors or acts that you have communicated clearly you are either not into or do not feel good about. This is not okay and will severely hurt your relationship if it continues.

8. Your partner watches TV or relaxes while you run around like crazy, cramming as much as you can in every minute of the evening—taking care of the house, kids, and so on. I honestly don't think there is any bigger turnoff.

THE GOOD SEX DIET: EAT MORE APHRODISIACS

Yes, it's true. Some foods are purported to perpetuate desire and can even make you feel sexier. Luckily, many of them are also good for you, so it doesn't hurt to give them a try. The following are some suggestions on great foods that will jump-start your libido:

- Avocados, known since ancient times as "the sensuous fruit," are high in omega-3 fatty acids, magnesium, and zinc, which are all important to a healthy body and sex drive.

- Figs are an excellent source of iron, magnesium, and zinc.

- Oysters are said to boost sexual vigor. They are high in zinc and omega-3 fatty acids, essentials for a healthy sex drive.

- Salmon is also loaded with omega-3s. If you're going to eat seafood, though, be sure to eat wild, not farmed, varieties. They're much better for you and won't have the antibiotics and hormones that farmed fish have.

- Foods that create warmth, such as spicy peppers and curry, are said to create desire. The same goes for foods that are smooth, rich, creamy, or exotic.

- Chocolate. Need I say more? Eating one ounce of dark chocolate daily boosts dopamine, the neurotransmitter that enables men and women to experience sexual pleasure. The darker the chocolate, the better.

- Limit caffeine and energy drinks that are full of sugar and other stimulants. They're an orgasm killer. Too much caffeine and other stimulants can create a strain on your adrenals, spiking and then quickly dropping serotonin, which makes you feel exhausted, anxious, and strung out. This is not the best condition to be in for a healthy sexual experience. The goal with good sex is being relaxed.

- Stop smoking! Nicotine reduces blood flow to the clitoris and penis and results in reduced sexual sensation and function. After only two cigarettes, studies show a significant decrease in the size of the main artery carrying blood to the sexual organs.

IMPROVE YOUR SEX LIFE WITH EXERCISE

You've heard all about the benefits of regular exercise in making you feel better, lose weight, get more sleep, and improve your quality of life, but on top of all this, exercise can also dramatically improve your sex life. This is yet another reason why it's so worth it to start engaging in some physical changes that will make you happier. After even a few weeks of regular exercise and improved fitness, you'll notice the benefits under the covers with more stamina, the desire to have sex more often, feeling more playful and fun, and increased flexibility and self-esteem. Bottom line: Active people have better sex drives.

- **Get on the cardio train.** Go to a gym, hit the streets in your walking or running shoes, jump on a bicycle, grab a jump rope, take a dance class, or do anything active five to seven days a week that increases your heart rate enough to break a sweat for a minimum of 10 minutes. Work up to 40 minutes, five days a week.

- **Stretch daily.** Keep your muscles from seizing up. Stretch every day, even if just for 15 minutes. Touch your toes and hold them, arch your back and hold it, and grab your shoulders with your hands and move your elbows together and hold the pose. Sit on a firm chair and, keeping your back straight, rest your right foot or ankle directly above your left knee. Then, lean forward with your back straight to stretch your right hip. Hold for at least 30 seconds. Then do the same to stretch your left hip.

- **Exercise your sex muscles.** Women, your PC (pubococcygeus) muscle needs a regular workout. If your goal is to reach peak performance with sex, you must exercise the muscles throughout your pelvis. Research shows that women with weak pelvic floor muscles are less likely to have orgasms than women with strong pelvic floor muscles. To locate this muscle, stick your finger into your vagina and close down on it. This is the PC muscle, and you should work it daily. Tightening this muscle, then releasing, and then tightening again promotes wonderful blood flow and is an easy and invisible exercise. Try doing it several times a day.

FAST TRACK TO BETTER SEX

You know the drill. What follows is a plan to quickly get your libido burning and reignite a healthy and fulfilling sex life. Let's get to it.

- Trouble achieving orgasm might be hormonal. First and foremost, if you have a healthy relationship with your mate and your sex drive is still rock bottom, get your hormones tested immediately. My sex drive finally improved after I got testosterone pellets inserted under my skin. Testosterone is essential for drive and orgasms. Trying to have a mind-blowing orgasm with no testosterone is like spitting into the wind, and it's way too much work. Other hormones that can cause a low libido are thyroid and estrogen. Fixing your hormones will also help fix vaginal dryness and pain during sex, and it will make your orgasms stronger. So you'll want to get this amended as soon as possible. The typical times that fluctuating hormones can negatively impact a woman's drive are

  - The week before menstruation—premenstrual syndrome

  - After giving birth—postpartum depression

  - During perimenopause—the 10–15 years before menopause

  - Menopause—after menstruation ceases and hormone production declines dramatically

- Think about sex. Let the anticipation build throughout the day. Regain the longing you had when you were dating or when you first married. Make it a point to touch your partner often, brushing up against him or her with a little extra oomph. Try sexting and talking about sex more often with your partner. In the morning, communicate about how excited you are for your time together that night. Express love and appreciation for each other. Give signals that you are going to do something new. If you don't feel like it, do it anyway. You can change your mind by changing your behavior. Focus on the benefits. The rewards will be worth every effort you put into it. Remember, a lot of sexual drive is mental.

- Add sex drive supplementation. L-arginine at a higher dose (5,000 mg) is not only effective for erectile problems but also useful for helping women have more efficient orgasms.

- Track your menstrual cycle (if you are not on hormone birth control). During the premenstrual phase, you will likely need twice the amount of foreplay to have an orgasm. So, start the foreplay on the couch and tell your partner why that is important. During the first 14 days of your cycle (day one is the first day of your period), you will be more turned on by a sexy novel or something new in the bedroom. During ovulation (midcycle), you will be able to have the best orgasm with less work.

- Get out of bed. A change in scenery is one of the best ways to keep a sense of novelty in your sex life. Make it comfortable for you or just encourage playing around before going to bed exhausted.

- Take a bath or read or watch something sexy on TV to relax your mind. You can even take or use something to relax, whether that be lavender, CBD oil, GABA, or anything that will help turn off your brain. Your brain *must* be disengaged to have good sex. So stop thinking about the laundry or the meeting you have at work tomorrow. Turn it off.

- Consider using another form of birth control if needed. I typically give my patients natural progesterone and testosterone when they use the hormone birth control methods, as they all cause testosterone and progesterone to drop off, leaving you feeling depressed and with little or no sex drive, and they can also compromise the frequency and intensity of orgasms. While I still prescribe birth control, I pay attention to the hormone levels of my patients when taking them. This helps alleviate the unnecessary marital problems that stem from a drop in libido.

- A great deal of research has been focused on the physical aspect of sex for women, but not nearly enough on the mental aspect. Male brains seemed to be focused on the physical stimulation during sex, but the key for women is deep relaxation and a lack of anxiety. Brain scans of women during sex show that the parts of the brain responsible for processing fear and anxiety start to relax more and more as they get closer to orgasm. As the female's anxiety and emotion are effectively closed down, orgasm occurs. Interesting, huh? Almost poetic. You really can't be thinking of anything else except how amazing it feels to be taken care of. Lie back and enjoy, ladies. It's the only way to have an orgasm.

- Make eye contact. Focus on making eye contact with your partner (not staring, of course). This can transfer sexual energy to each other, and for men it is a major turn-on.

- Sleep, baby, sleep! More/better sleep leads to more/better sex.

- Check your medications. Low sex drive is a common side effect of birth control pills, antidepressants, tranquilizers, high blood pressure pills, and other medications. Diabetes, and the medications prescribed to treat it, can also reduce sexual function.

- Consider replaying some of the things you did when you first got together with your partner. Keep your clothes on longer, taking one item off at a time, and above all, take your time. It heightens the oxytocin levels to drag out the anticipation a little more. Teach your partner to wait. Consider not waiting to get into bed for anything to happen—the "need you now" urgency will make your session even hotter.

- Send sexy or suggestive messages throughout the day. Keeping your thoughts on sex will pay off that night. This is more for the sake of better sex for women, as women need to be focused on sex throughout the day more than men to achieve a heightened sex drive.

- Consider a massage. Get the oil out and have your partner rub the areas on your body that are most sensual to you—lower back, inner thighs, outer breasts, whatever feels good. Tell your partner you will be more interested in sex if you are massaged first. (This will help you relax and get you unwound from the day.)

- Love your naked body. Truly one of the downers for sexual satisfaction is a woman not loving her body. Seeing yourself as strong and sexy is important in order to have satisfying sex. There are numerous ways to get your self-love back on track and improve the way you feel about yourself. If you are feeling ugly, unhealthy, unattractive, and weak, then it's time for some self-work. Ironically, the most powerful, successful, amazing women I have ever met tend to hate their bodies. We need to think enough about ourselves to change this. Plus, when we like ourselves, we are more attractive to others.

- Try a new position. Many couples get into certain habits in the bedroom that they know make their partner happy. Consider instead trying new things that will keep the excitement and anticipation elevated.

- The lips are packed with nerve endings, 100 times more powerful than the fingertips. So please kiss, kiss, kiss—it really makes sex more powerful.

- Buy a present for yourself. Consider looking at a Victoria's Secret catalog or a website with your partner and selecting a couple of sexy items to purchase that you both like.

- Try some orgasm cream. I have long prescribed a cream in my office that is a combination of Viagra, aminophylline, and L-arginine. This is applied to the clitoral and vaginal opening to dilate the blood vessels, bring in more blood flow, and voilà, a great orgasm. It's a simple approach that helps fire things up more!

- Get yourself ready for sex. Make a sexy playlist that you both love that will put you in the mood. Consider going to bed to relax before your partner climbs in so that you are ready and relaxed. This will greatly help your ability to climax.

- Try silent sex. Sorry, guys, we women don't typically need a lot of talking. We are trying to focus on relaxing. Sex can be very exciting with silence rather than full volume. Pay attention to the physical cues and facial expressions and see what happens. It's incredible how connected you can feel without words.

- Communicate with your partner. You need to tell them what you need, what you like, and what you don't like. If your partner is a man, you must remember that men are simple creatures, and they usually just want to please you, so tell them how you feel and what you need.

- Go to bed earlier. Don't go to bed so exhausted. Try to use your daytime hours more wisely to get the maximum effect of what you need. Studies show there is a link between lack of sleep and disinterest in sex. Good sex requires rest; otherwise, it will not be worth the effort.

- And last but certainly not least, get rid of distractions. Please put away your cell phones, computers, and any other work-related items at least an hour before bed to mentally prepare yourself for good sex. Remember, screen or work time before bed can stress you out, but women need maximum relaxation and no anxiety to have good orgasms, and this only gets trickier the older you get. Get out of your head and start winding down early if you want to have fulfilling sex.

In summary, sexual satisfaction plays a big role in women's success, whether you're with someone you love or taking matters into your own hands, you need to be sexually satisfied regularly in order to be at your best. This outlet is necessary for driven women, and we need to acknowledge how much all of our relationships are improved because of it. Our bodies are built for this, and women should be proud of the fact that we have this special way to reset at our disposal.

Sex Drive Success Story

Kelly came to my office in tears several years ago. She hated that her sex drive was in the tank, along with her ability to have an orgasm like she used to. Her relationship with her husband was amazing. They were great partners and friends, but she literally had no interest in sex, and it was starting to become an issue.

She was a successful financial analyst and loved her work and family. From the outside, she had it all. She was 48 years old and vibrant. She had a strong body, a healthy mind-set, had no emotional issues, and from what I could initially tell, had no other reason for a poor sex drive and inability to have an orgasm except for debunked hormones.

After some preliminary testing, it was evident that her testosterone was as low as it could go. She had zero, zilch, nada. Obviously, this was the thing we had to fix first and foremost. But things are rarely that simple. I explained that because it had been years of negative feedback with an inability to have an orgasm that these neurological patterns often become deep seated, and it takes time for the correct responses to reintegrate in the brain. Kelly was in it for the long haul, though, and together we came up with a strategy to get her back on track.

Her game plan included the following:

- Immediately starting testosterone therapy to replace what she had lost

- Beginning meditation on sex to help rewire her brain

- Engaging her husband in a sex-rehab plan

- Boosting her testosterone before sex with a topical application to the clitoral area

I had her start testosterone therapy and engage with her husband in a sex rehab plan that included meditation and a topical testosterone cream. This really got the party started. The testosterone therapy turned her world around. In only two weeks, her sexual desire came back in full force, and not too long after that she began to feel like her old self again. Kelly also worked on some self-esteem issues over time and learned to communicate better sexually with her husband, and now, three years later, they are still going strong.

9

Brilliant Energy: Start Your Engines

"Become more aware of what is really worth your energy."

—*UNKNOWN*

In this chapter you will learn how to recognize the insidious onset of exhaustion and turn it around. Take a minute—if you can spare the energy—and fill out this quiz to find your level of exhaustion.

QUIZ: ARE YOU EXHAUSTED?

1. Do you have trouble getting up in the morning? Y/N
2. Do you rely on a cup of coffee to get you going in the morning? Y/N
3. Do you feel tired all the time? Y/N
4. Do you often feel foggy, fuzzy, flat, or dull? Y/N
5. Do you have trouble concentrating or remembering things? Y/N
6. Do you need artificial stimulants or medication to wake you up? Y/N
7. Do you hit the wall in the afternoon? Y/N

8. Are you wiped out after a significant emotionally charged incident? Y/N

9. Do you bruise easily or get dizzy when you stand up quickly? Y/N

10. Do you have trouble sleeping deeply at night? Y/N

11. Do you use sugar or caffeine as a pick-me-up throughout the day? Y/N

12. Are you often irritable or angry, for no apparent reason? Y/N

13. Do your moods seem to go up and down for no apparent reason? Y/N

14. Are your mood swings often relieved by food, especially sweets? Y/N

15. Is your diet low in protein and high in carbohydrates? Y/N

16. Do you find yourself operating from crisis to crisis? Y/N

17. Are you drawn to thrills, danger, or drama in your life? Y/N

Total number of yes answers: ＿＿＿＿＿＿＿

Less than 5 yes answers: Who are you, Wonder Woman? You're probably doing fine; however, be careful, because fatigue creeps in with bad habits on board.

5–10 yes answers: Shocker, you're human. This means your energy is compromised, and you need to take steps to understand what's happening in your body and how to make healthier choices to ultimately improve your energy naturally.

More than 10 yes answers: I'm going to be real with you: You may be seriously hooked on stimulants, and it's affecting your mental and physical health. It's important for you to take yourself off them.

....

Let's face it, being a modern woman is *hard*, and dealing with exhaustion will not make it any easier. So what's tapping your energy and leading to exhaustion? Why do we so often feel tired for no real reason? This is a critical question to address because, trust me, it's hard to have it all when the only things you want by 3:00 p.m. are a glass of rosé and a nap.

Yet the fact is millions of women are walking around exhausted and have no idea why. You may not even realize how tired you are because you have been tired for so long now. Fatigue can take many forms and can stem from literally hundreds of reasons. It could be something as simple as an iron deficiency, not sleeping deeply enough, or a borderline low thyroid, but the sad fact is that usually several things are happening at the same time, creating an energy drain.

THE CAUSES OF FATIGUE

At this point, it shouldn't surprise you to hear that fatigue is the number-one reason women and men seek help at our Peak Medical Clinic practices, and it is the basis of the vast majority of visits to other medical offices. Fatigue and exhaustion are by far the most prevalent medical issues plaguing modern society. This is because there are hundreds of reasons for fatigue that medical professionals often dismiss or chalk up to stress and depression. In the traditional medical office, it is uncommon that a woman would get a thorough evaluation of fatigue that addressed more than the most obvious medical issues. Delving deep into the potential underlying roots of the problem by looking at diet, sleep, stress, female hormone balance, emotional and mental stress, nutrients, gut health, autoimmune disorders, and possible medication or food sensitivities is not typically something offered to women when they have fatigue issues. But, of course, that's why you're reading this book.

In our clinics, the first and most obvious place to start in identifying where the energy drain is coming from is to look at the daily habits of each patient, because even the best medical care can be thwarted by an addiction to sugar. In conjunction with this, we perform blood tests to look at adrenal, thyroid, and ovarian hormones; nutrient levels; brain chemical levels; and other markers for autoimmune disorders as well as the basic chemistries of the body. We also look at gut health to ensure nothing is reducing absorption of vitamins and nutrients within the gut, as well as food sensitivities that are causing body inflammation, zapping the energy stores.

When working with women, I explain there are certain basics of fatigue management that must be kept sacred to sustain energy as you age. If only one of these basics is dropped, a highly stressed woman is bound to end up with exhaustion at some point. It's a cross to bear as a hardworking woman, no doubt, but categorizing the fatigue problems into areas makes it a little easier to digest and helps women find their way back to vibrant energy every day.

The main areas I see that seem to be the source of fatigue in women today are the following:

1. Self-neglect or poor lifestyle habits

2. Medical issues

3. Excessive emotional baggage

4. Nutrient and hormone deficiencies

Self-Neglect or Poor Lifestyle Habits

It should come as no surprise that, these days, poor habits are the main cause of fatigue in women. This includes your diet, your sleep habits, your schedule… everything. Your food will either heal you or kill you. If you are consistently eating foods high in sugar and carbohydrates, you will feel bad. If you run yourself into the ground and do not give yourself a break during the day, you will hit a wall in the afternoon. If you have interrupted sleep or not enough sleep, you will be lacking in zest and stamina.

As ironic as it may sound, the fundamental key to achieving high energy is to do what I call "daily work." Plan ahead, eat well and timely, quiet your brain daily, exercise, sleep deeply, and be conscious of when you need to stop working to give your body rest. These are the basics. Do them every day. And when you get off track, get your ass back in gear and begin again. There's no shame in stumbling on the path to success, but you cannot, I repeat, *cannot* keep going at the pace you want to go with good energy, brain function, mood, and clarity without practicing the basics. They must be a religion to you.

Here are some super simple self-care basics that you can look out for and implement into your daily life right now.

DIET

1. Drink plenty of water. This seems pretty elementary, but dehydration is strongly linked to fatigue. Medical experts estimate that something as low as a 2 percent fluid loss can have a significant impact on our energy levels. This is because this loss of fluid causes a visible reduction in blood volume. Dehydration makes our blood pump less efficiently, restricting oxygen and nutrients from getting to our muscles and organs. And, no, wine does not count as hydration.

2. Don't eat a breakfast high in sugar. This is such a common problem for working women. Eating energy zappers like donuts, bagels, or muffins with juice will only set you up for a sluggish, uphill battle kind of day. You might as well take a sleeping pill first thing in the morning.

3. Stay away from junk food. This is a surefire way of killing your system and draining any remaining energy you have. As insane as it sounds, I honestly believe many people think they can go weeks without eating veggies and not pay a price. The reality is that eat-

ing a low-nutrient diet can cause exhaustion and will give you no help in the energy department. On the contrary, in fact; junk foods are typically high on the glycemic scale, which means they raise your glucose and set us up for a system crash, leaving you feeling more tired than you did before you reached for the "fatigue fix."

4. Don't drink alcohol before bed. I know, I know—but hear me out! Alcohol before bed creates poor sleep patterns and interrupts your restorative rest. The kind of sleep you get after having several drinks can wake you up during the night and keep you from getting back to sleep, leaving you exhausted in the morning.

5. Make sure you get enough iron. Iron deficiency seems to be a problem that is on the rise. This is likely due to poor diet. Vegans are particularly susceptible to becoming anemic because of the lack of B-12 and iron in their diets. Even if you're a lifelong carnivore like my husband, it's still something you should watch out for. Iron deficiency can cause weakness, exhaustion, dark circles under the eyes, increased bruising, compromised concentration, and dizziness upon standing. With less iron in our blood, the amount of oxygen that can get to the muscles and cells in the body is reduced. And no oxygen means no energy.

EXERCISE

1. Don't skip workouts. Not working out can cause fatigue. And don't worry, it's perfectly normal to feel personally betrayed by your body after hearing that fact. The key to addressing this (if necessary) is to find a shorter period of time to work out so you can at least get in some exercise to increase the oxygen flow to your brain and muscles to sustain your energy.

2. You lose muscle mass with age. The loss of muscle mass (the only metabolically active part of our body) with age reduces strength and energy and creates a loss of overall metabolism. As we age, we lose 1–3 percent of our muscle mass annually, which reduces our metabolism, so we must continue to build and restore our muscle mass or our metabolism will drop, causing fatigue, weight gain, and overall lowered stamina.

MEDITATION AND MENTAL DOWNTIME

Taking a few minutes during the day to clear your mind is a must. Some of you may be rolling your eyes at the idea, but mental rest is as important as physical rest. This practice is needed to open up space for creativity, ideas, solutions, answers, and (of course) genius thoughts. The outlet created from daily meditation and centering will allow you to see things differently and keep you open mentally and emotionally. I like to call it "clearing the mechanism." The mechanism to be cleared, of course, is your cluttered-up, ransacked, overfilled brain. If you never clear the mechanism, you will be unable to focus, concentrate, or react to stressful situations in the most positive way.

Try meditation or frequent conscious mental clearing. You can clear your mind daily by breathing deeply and focusing on releasing thoughts of anxiety and worry, with your eyes closed. Try this at set times during the day, and tie it to something else you know you'll do—like taking a restroom break—so you remember to practice it.

SLEEP

Sleep, next to diet, may be the most important habit for recovering from fatigue and gaining more energy. Even if you have a physical condition that causes fatigue, sleep is still considered necessary for recovery. Your body needs everything in balance to function properly, so losing rest and not getting restorative sleep can contribute to hormonal imbalances that will make you even more fatigued.

While you sleep, your body makes necessary hormones that are vital for energy. This is why you need seven to eight good hours of sleep each night—and more if you are under high stress or dealing with intense emotional issues. Your entire nervous system will reboot nightly with enough sleep, which is, frankly, something of a miracle. But if your sleep is constantly compromised, your body will let you know—you'll be exhausted. Even if you think you are getting enough sleep on paper, you might not be for the level of stress you are under. So, if you are still feeling tired after a good seven or eight hours of sleep, you may need to go to bed a little earlier to get in some additional sleep time to help you get a more complete reboot. Your body will thank you.

Medical Issues

Many medical problems and conditions cause fatigue and exhaustion, and if the worrisome issues have been ruled out, you might consider getting the following tested to optimize energy if you are still having problems:

LOW IRON

I've said it before and I'll say it again: Anemia is a major cause of fatigue. Red blood cells deliver oxygen to your organs, which keeps them functioning optimally. Diagnosing and fixing low iron can significantly help fatigue. This can also help fix your gut balance so you can better absorb the iron from your food and supplements via the gut, which will help correct the anemia. Diagnosing and treating excessive yeast in the gut will help resolve exhaustion. This will also help improve the absorption of other nutrients and vitamins. Fixing low ferritin will also help to support the thyroid gland and circulating thyroid levels.

DEPRESSION AND ANXIETY

Some women say that no matter how much sleep they get, they are still exhausted. They feel unmotivated and unable to get through their daily tasks. In cases like these, the problem may lie not with the body, but the brain. Depression and anxiety can be serious underlying causes of fatigue. The stress hormone cortisol contributes to your mood, and when it is low it can lead to other hormone disruptions that not only cause fatigue but also depression and anxiety, leading to more fatigue. In this case, though, instead of treating the fatigue directly, it is important to treat depression so we are not simply putting a Band-Aid on the problem.

AUTOIMMUNE SYNDROMES

Autoimmune disorders are complicated and on the rise.[34] Although I can't tell you what exactly has caused the increase, as there are numerous precursors to these disorders, I can tell you that I have diagnosed more autoimmune disorders in the last year than the previous five years combined. Autoimmune disorders create significant inflammation. This inflammation is one of the leading causes of fatigue today. Chronic fatigue syndrome is chief among these. It is a debilitating and complex disorder characterized by fatigue that lasts more than six months, and it is not improved by resting; physical and emotional stress make it worse. There are many subtypes of chronic fatigue, and all autoimmune disorders have a significant fatigue component.

Some of the subtypes of chronic fatigue are the following:

- Post-exertional malaise is characterized by extreme weakness and discomfort after minimal amounts of activity.

34   Monika Hybenova, Pavlina Hrda, Jarmila Procházková, Vera Stejskal, and Ivan Sterzl, "The Role of Environmental Factors in Autoimmune Thyroiditis," *Neuroendocrinology Letters* 31, no.3 (2010) 283–289, https://www.ncbi.nlm.nih.gov/pubmed/20588228.

- Wired fatigue causes a woman to feel overly stimulated combined with extreme lack of energy.

- Brain fog fatigue is characterized by mental impairment, confusion, and an inability to function in daily activities due to disorientation.

- Flu-like fatigue causes feelings of weakness and flu-like symptoms with sore glands and fevers.

- Energy fatigue creates a feeling of heaviness and immobilization without energy to do any daily tasks. Often women are housebound with this type of fatigue.

HYPOTHYROIDISM

Thyroid dysfunction can be hereditary, and so can autoimmune disorders of the thyroid. You cannot afford to lack optimal circulating thyroid hormones. And simply because you don't have a goiter the size of a grapefruit doesn't mean your thyroid is perfectly healthy. Even a suboptimal thyroid can be a problem. (In my opinion, a suboptimal thyroid should be treated in the presence of exhaustion or symptoms of low thyroid.) Blood levels of thyroid T3 and T4 should be in the mid to upper end of the ideal range.

Unstable or Low Cortisol Levels

With extreme stress over time, the adrenals begin to underproduce cortisol to conserve energy and give you time to help manage stress. The problem is that low cortisol can make you as though like you're running a marathon every day. It is one of the most exhausting things you can experience. In addition, the high inflammatory response, insulin resistance, glucose instability, interrupted sleep patterns, and low testosterone that all are associated with imbalanced stress hormones further ransack the energy stores.

Suboptimal Testosterone and Estradiol Levels

Periods of hormonal imbalance can be triggered for women at certain hormonal transitions, such as during postpartum, PMS, perimenopause, and menopause. This type of exhaustion can be debilitating. It feels as though someone slowly removed your ability to manage your daily functioning, causing you to have a reduced ability to tolerate stress and the emotional capacity to put up with it.

In addition, many other medical conditions lead to fatigue. However, for most high-stressed women, this is where I would begin zoning in on their potential energy zappers.

Excessive Emotional Baggage

This area is so broad and so significant that it's a bit daunting to even touch on. That said, it is absolutely something that needs addressing on your journey to overcoming burnout, so stick with me.

I have personally encountered the fatigue that comes from excessive emotional upheaval. Most women never have the opportunity to truly understand or learn to connect the dots of exhaustion and emotional upset. Our lives are moving at such a rapid pace that we don't even take the time to see it and acknowledge it, let alone correct it.

In addition, we are quickly becoming a society that is moving away from emotion, so we mostly move on or take a pill to not feel anything, without any resolution to the significant emotional events that we encounter. Worse still, we often engage in the very mental and emotional activities that worsen our fatigue. These include, but are not limited to, replaying a problem or conversation over and over in our head without the ability to turn it off or come back to reality; constantly worrying about people, situations, or events that likely will never happen; and regurgitating a stressful situation over and over to multiple people so that by the second or third time saying it, you are more wound up than ever.

Unless you are some sort of saint, we all get stuck in this kind of behavior, and it is simply not healthy.

Why do we do this? Is it for a sense of control? Maybe it gives us time to focus on something else, because the other 1,000 things we have to think about and process are not enough? (Yeah, right.) Regardless of the reasons, I've made a list of the emotional energy killers of biggest concern. Watch out for worry and emotional baggage.

WORRY

This is a big one. We habitually sweat the small stuff, which makes us physically and emotionally exhausted. Sometimes, we even lose sight of what is small and what is significant. We worry too much about the smallest things to attain a sense of control. Meanwhile, our energy levels plummet.

Sometimes, we are in a situation that is negative at work, at home, or with family members we can't get away from. The negativity and resentment these situations breed are a surefire way to achieve fatigue. Worrying too much has a significant detrimental effect on your physical health. It can leave you mentally and physically exhausted, negatively affect hormone and brain chemical levels, and interrupt sleep patterns. It can also cause all sorts of chronic body pain, gut disorders, and headaches. In other words, constant worry can physically make you sick. When I see a patient with excessive worry, I always tell them, "Be careful what you worry about; it just may come true." Wherever your mind goes, there also goes your body and life.

EMOTIONAL BAGGAGE

We all carry emotional baggage to varying degrees—painful childhood memories, grief over the loss of a loved one, the devastation of a marriage or relationship breakup, rejection, betrayal, hardship, failure, shame, longing, guilt, loss of self-esteem, or sorrow. Or even all of the above.

It's easier for most of us to give in to the assumption that we can move quickly beyond the emotions of anger, resentment, guilt, grief, or negativity to avoid pain and request medication to numb us, so we don't have to feel or face it. The reality is that the actual incident or emotional trauma is not the worst thing; the worst thing is not working through it. So it lingers, affecting nearly every aspect of our emotional and physical health for years to come. Trust me: Burying it never works.

What does this have to do with fatigue? It turns out, quite a lot. It takes more effort and energy to keep pain in your body than it does to confront it and release it. The stress of shutting out emotions takes its toll on us physically, and the longer we live with low energy caused by unresolved or unmanaged emotions, the more it begins to feel normal. Fortunately, most women at some point will realize they don't feel well and want to find a way to get help.

Powerful emotions, such as pain, fear, grief, disappointment, panic, anxiety, anger, and longing, can shock your body, creating inflammation along your neural pathways. This disrupts your body's natural energy flow and leads to fatigue and pain. Condensed molecules from the breath exhaled during verbal expressions of anger, hatred, and jealousy contain toxins that get stored in your body over time, creating a huge toxic mess.

Suppressing emotions also uses up a lot of energy that should be used for vital functions. Negative emotions can tax your spleen, liver, and adrenal glands and use up nutrients the body needs to sustain itself. The result is fatigue, autoimmune disorders, and a loss of zest for life. Energy has to move. If an emotion isn't expressed, then it will be suppressed internally, feeding off your energy like a parasite.

Nutrient and Hormone Deficiencies

Identifying underlying nutrient deficiencies and swiftly fixing them can be one of the most efficient ways of treating chronic fatigue. A simple blood test can be performed to look at nutrient levels, and then an optimal nutrition and supplement plan can be given based on these results. This can even be repeated several times a year if needed to ensure you're getting optimal nutrition. Some of the nutrients most closely tied to energy are the following:

- Vitamin D

- Zinc

- Magnesium

- B vitamins

- Coenzyme Q10

- L-tyrosine

- *Rhodiola rosea*

VITAMIN D

Most women should be on a high dosage of vitamin D3. It's a tiny pill, but its benefits are staggering. This vitamin can also be gathered via the sun during certain times of the year for most geographical areas. Don't break out the tanning lotion just yet, though. The concern with trying to get vitamin D from the sun is that many women do not absorb enough through their skin to achieve an optimal level of 60–80 ng/ml. And if you stay out too long, you risk UV damage, which comes with its own host of problems. Nonetheless, getting proper levels of this nutrient is essential, as vitamin D not only dramatically increases energy, but it also improves mood, concentration, endurance, the immune system, and lower body strength.

ZINC

Among all the minerals found in the human body, zinc remains one that few people outside the medical and scientific community truly understand. Fatigue sufferers should be especially cognizant of the vital nature of the body's zinc supply and the fatigue and other symptoms that can accompany zinc deficiency.

What's most important to understand is that zinc is essential if vitamins are to be able to do their jobs. It exists in some small quantity in virtually all of the body's cells and carries with it hundreds of the enzymes the body needs to make use of the other vitamins you consume.

In other words, zinc doesn't do much for your body directly, but it helps other things that your body needs work faster and more efficiently. Without the right levels of this mineral, your cells are unable to properly utilize the nutrients provided by your consumption of food, leaving you with a disrupted capacity for energy production. That obviously leads to the type of energy drop that can result in severe fatigue. Zinc is also excellent for improving hormone balance and promoting testosterone and natural energy for men and women, and you definitely want to make sure you're getting enough of it every day.

MAGNESIUM

Give me a large, double shot, no foam magnesium latte please! One of the primary roles of magnesium in energy production is its partnership with ATP (adenosine triphosphate), the energy "currency" of the cell. In fact, ATP *needs* to be partnered with magnesium to be biologically active. This ATP complex acts as a sort of chemical battery, powering numerous functions and processes, including our mitochondria's ability to create more ATP out of food energy. Optimal magnesium is also important for muscle and bone support and improving the quality of sleep at night. For best results, take this supplement at bedtime.

B VITAMINS

B vitamins are the body's powerhouse of energy, but more than that they are integral to maintaining mental well-being. They are precursors to our brain chemicals, and with high dosages one can easily turn around depression, anxiety, and chronic fatigue. B vitamins are often depleted during stress and can be reduced through a poor diet or medications you are taking that inhibit your body's absorption of these vitamins.

Vitamin B1 (thiamine) supports mental well-being and mood, vitamin B2 (riboflavin) helps reduce oxidative stress (and therefore tiredness), vitamin B3 (niacin) has been shown to be effective in supporting brain functions, and vitamin B5 (pantothenic acid) helps support important neurotransmitters (brain chemicals). Then, there's vitamin B6 (pyridoxine hydrochloride), which plays a part in reducing fatigue and strengthening immunity, even when you're under stress, and vitamin B8 (inositol), which helps nerve signals communicate.

COENZYME Q10

You've probably heard of this one in the headline of some nutrition article or featured in a banner ad on Facebook, but what exactly is CoQ10? Often called the miracle nutrient or the universal antioxidant, CoQ10 exists in the mitochondria, which are the tiny energy centers in each of our cells. Inside of these little powerhouses, not only does CoQ10 scavenge and destroy free radicals that cause cardiovascular problems and heart disease, but it also sparks energy production in every cell of your body, including the heart.

Unsurprisingly, then, one of the major benefits of having proper levels of CoQ10 is improved energy. The heart is one of the few organs in the body that functions continuously, without resting. Therefore, the heart muscle (myocardium) requires the largest level of energetic support of any organ in your body. In fact, any condition that causes a decrease in CoQ10 can impair the energetic capacity of the heart, leaving the tissues more susceptible to free radical attack. When your body is low on CoQ10, you will feel run down. Unfortunately, many people write off this feeling as a sign of getting old. They never realize that the real cause of the problem is a CoQ10 deficiency.

L-TYROSINE

L-tyrosine is an amino acid that can counteract stress before it happens. Yep, you read that right: When taken before an event that's anticipated to be stressful, it can head off stress hormones at the pass. How? Well, when we're stressed, our bodies secrete a lot of the neurotransmitters adrenaline and dopamine, which help keep the typical symptoms of stress at bay. But we've only got a finite amount of those two chemicals, so when we run out of them, that's when we experience symptoms of stress, like fatigue, sweatiness, and a serious decrease in motivation and attention. No fun, right? That's why it can be helpful to make sure there's plenty of L-tyrosine in the blood, since it helps the body produce adrenaline and dopamine and thereby protects us from the effects of stress. It's ideal to take 500–2,000 milligrams of L-tyrosine an hour before the stressful event is supposed to occur, or—if your entire life is a stressful event—once to twice daily, preferably on an empty stomach.

RHODIOLA ROSEA

Rhodiola rosea is another adaptogen that can help desensitize someone to a stressful event before it happens. Derived from an herb that grows in the chillier parts of Northern Europe, rhodiola is safe and effective at treating metabolic burnout, and there's some evidence that it's effective at combating mild depression and improving cognition, to boot.

While researchers aren't completely sure how the herb works, they do know that it helps maintain proper serotonin levels in the brain, which can affect our moods and hormones—but further research is needed to determine exactly how this adaptogen functions in our bodies. In any event, rhodiola is thought to be safe and effective and can even be taken once a day without any decrease in effectiveness.

FATIGUE TRIGGERS

Most women who come to my office complain of some level of fatigue. For some, this is a new development, but most have significant exhaustion that has surfaced over a longer period of time. In order to get to the bottom of what is happening and to help uncover the underlying issues or precursors of fatigue, I give them a questionnaire that looks at contributing factors to fatigue. This helps to not only give me a clue how to treat them, but it is also a tool to help them see what little things are tapping their energy stores daily, which over time can be quite damaging.

To address your personal energy crisis and repair the elements that are depleting your vitality, it's important to be sensitive to the specific messages your body is sending you. You need to listen closely to what your exhaustion is telling you. Otherwise, how can you possibly expect to undo the damage and restore your vigor to healthier levels? It's not enough to recognize that your energy balance is out of whack. You also need to figure out *why* it's off-kilter.

The first step toward breaking the exhaustion cycle is to identify and understand what is zapping your energy and contributing to your profound sense of fatigue. Then, and only then, can you begin to take steps to revitalize and reclaim your energy and well-being. So, let's start that identification process by answering the following questions:

WHAT'S CONTRIBUTING TO YOUR EXHAUSTION?

1. Is your fatigue worse first thing in the morning, midday, late after-noon, or evening?

2. Do you have trouble falling asleep or staying asleep?

3. Do you skip on sleep to get more done in the evenings?

4. Do you skip breakfast or go longer than four hours without eating during the day?

5. Do you drink eight glasses of water per day?

6. Do you eat sugar or flour or starches to boost your energy during the day? Are you a real carb lover?

7. Is your diet low in protein? Do you have protein with each meal?

8. Do you crave sugar or salt daily?

9. Would you consider yourself overly stressed most of the day or excessively hurried?

10. Do you feel depressed, down, or anxious daily?

11. Do you feel more exhausted after a stressful incident, as if you were hit by a Mack Truck?

12. Do you find yourself holding your breath when driving, during stressful times of the day, or when you are working on your computer?

13. Is it hard for you to turn off the work and shut your eyes to relax when it feels like you're under too much stress?

14. Do you get daily exercise or times when you are able to walk and stretch throughout the day?

15. Do you carve out at least ten minutes daily to decompress and breathe while thinking about nothing?

16. Do you find yourself worrying about your job, family, finances, or other issues more than three times during the day?

17. Do you spend your downtime trying to recover from your stressful week?

18. Do you spend time engaging in hobbies or spending time with friends doing fun things to recharge?

19. Do you drink alcohol to get yourself relaxed most nights?

20. Do you need caffeine to keep you going daily?

21. Do you wish you had more control of your life and wish you could experience fewer demands and stress daily?

If you answered all of these questions honestly, odds are you've identified a few stress issues you need to work on. Now that you have pinpointed some habits or triggers that might not be serving you well for energy, consider making note of these things and begin making some changes for the better. You know what the problems are. Now we have to address them. The following fast-track plan will help.

FAST-TRACK PLAN: IMPROVING YOUR ENERGY LEVELS

Sleep

- First and foremost, optimize all hormone levels. Nearly all hormones have something to do with sleep, and low levels or imbalanced hormones can interrupt or rob you of the one thing that helps you recover every 24 hours. Make sure to ask for hormone testing to evaluate the female hormones (specifically testosterone, thyroid, and cortisol) and shoot for upper ranges of optimal levels.

- Take sleep supplements if needed (see Appendix D).

- Consider taking supplements to recalibrate your cortisol rhythm (which should be higher during the day for energy and focus, and dead low at night for deep, restful, mindless sleep).

- Make sure the room you sleep in is cool, pitch dark, and dead quiet. Remove noisy people and animals if possible.

Diet

FOODS FOR ENERGY

- Eat protein at each meal for glucose regulation.

- Eat high-fiber, complex carbohydrate foods—foods that are higher in fiber slow the release of sugar in the system and will keep you satisfied longer with your appetite, resulting in a more balanced release of energy over time.

- Do not have sugar on an empty stomach (including sugary drinks).

- Consider drinking more coconut water. It is a natural electrolyte replacement.

- Eat nuts and seeds. Almonds, walnuts, hazelnuts, and cashews help regulate the release of energy supplied by fats and carbohydrates. The amino acids that make up the protein in nuts will boost neurotransmitters that will enhance mood and alertness. (Plus, chewing nuts reduces stress by stimulating the pressure receptors in the upper roof of the mouth, inducing calmness.) Seeds such as chia seeds are also excellent sources of omega-3 fatty acids, protein, fiber, and antioxidants. They contain higher amounts of B vitamins and calcium, which help rein in the stress cycle.

- Beans and lentils are rich in iron and vitamin C. These foods can help support low levels of iron and more effectively transport oxygen to the cells throughout your body.

- Blueberries are considered a superfood and are packed with key nutrients. They are rich in antioxidants, high in fiber, and have lots of vitamin C, which is vital for energy and brain function.

- Spinach is rich in magnesium, which is necessary for the production of adenosine triphosphate (ATP) energy. It is also rich in potassium, which helps transport nutrients to your cells for energy. Supporting magnesium and potassium can help prevent muscle weakness.

- Consume more iron-rich foods, such as lean beef, kidney beans, tofu, eggs, dark leafy veggies, and nuts. Consuming vitamin C can help you better absorb iron-rich foods. So, pair your steak and kale at dinner with an orange or grapefruit the next time you feel run down.

- Hydrate, hydrate, hydrate. A dehydrated body functions less efficiently.

- Be careful not to overdo caffeine. Energy drinks or coffee in excess can cause you to feel anxious, will overwork your heart, make you irritable, and affect your energy and performance.

- Don't overeat. Large meals, especially at lunch, will cause an afternoon slump. Eating less is always better for your energy. Ideally, try to not eat more than 400–600 calories per meal.

SUPPLEMENTS

If you have had nutrient testing done, follow these guidelines for replacement:

- Start a high-dose B complex supplement (sublingual preparations work great).

- Consider nutrient IVs or nutrient shots at your medical office that offers them.

- Consume 2,000–4,000 mg of vitamin C powder in the morning and afternoon in your water bottle to significantly reduce fatigue.

- Take high-dose vitamin D3 to optimize your blood level to 60–80 ng/ml.

- Incorporate amino acid supplements into your diet if you don't eat enough protein.

- If you need help with focus and stamina, try the amino acid L-tyrosine.

MEDITATION AND PRACTICING POSITIVE HABITS

- Try to devote at least ten minutes per day to breathing from your belly with your eyes closed, attempting to turn off your brain. Consider walking, meditations with exercise, or guided meditations as you go to sleep or first thing in the morning. This is a great way to start your day off right.

- Find five to six affirmations, and post them as many places as possible. Change them out monthly. These will serve as reminders to help correct negative thinking and abusive talk (especially about yourself or others) and will serve as excellent encouragement that will keep your spirits—and therefore your energy—up.

- Unclutter your environment, whether it is home or work. A messy environment restricts your ability to think clearly and makes you feel overwhelmed, as though you are unable to escape stress. A neat, organized space will make you feel efficient, relieve stress, and keep your energy levels up.

TESTING

I strongly encourage you to have an expert in the area of hormone balance test your levels. I promise that if you see someone knowledgeable in this field, it will be the best time and money spent to fix underlying imbalances creating the exhaustion.

- Hormones: estradiol, testosterone, and progesterone all done in the second half of the cycle (day 17–22 if menstruating)

- Thyroid: reverse T3, TSH, free T3, free T4, and thyroid antibodies

- Adrenal: pregnenolone, DHEA, and cortisol (in the a.m.)

- Ferritin (should be above 50 ng/ml)

- Complete metabolic panel (electrolytes, glucose, kidney, and liver enzymes)

- Complete blood count

- Food allergy testing (blood)

- Nutrient testing (blood)

- Bowel testing for candida and other pathogens

- Heavy metal testing

EMOTIONAL CARE

- Sometimes, medical care won't be enough. Studies show that as much as 80 percent of fatigue is caused from psychological factors. This means you should take steps to assess your level of psychological stress. Where is it coming from? Can you limit it? Can you move away from it? Does it serve a purpose in your life?

- Practice relaxation training. Persistent anxiety will kill your life energy. To combat this, switch off the adrenaline and move your body into the rest and relax mode during the day by breathing and taking a ten-minute walk while allowing your body to recover. Try to take a time out when you feel your body starting to get intensely tight.

- Remove negative people from your inner circle. Don't worry about them. Chances are they will likely find someone else they can bring down.

- Write down three negative emotions that you are continuing to struggle with that keep raising their ugly head throughout your week. Begin acknowledging these signs and reactions, and meditate on changing them. Walk along a beach or outside with bare feet, consider Reiki or reflexology treatment, and consider taking Epsom salt baths. Increase your physical activity, and start smiling more to combat negative emotions.

- Find at least three people to be in your tribe that support you, make you laugh, will keep you accountable, and will tell you when you are falling out of line with your self-care.

- Finally, and perhaps most importantly: Have fun and laugh at least once a day.

CURING THE AFTERNOON SLUMP

- The natural rhythm of the body is to start to wind down after 2:00 p.m. This is normal and part of the way we are wired. Taking a walk in the afternoon, removing yourself from hours of staring at a computer, and giving yourself a mental break will all help lift you out of this slump. Some other things you can do include the following:

- Eat a combination of protein and carbohydrates. Something like a lettuce-wrapped tuna sandwich will help power you up for hours.

- Eat an apple every afternoon. (This really works.)

- Add lemon to your water bottle for cleansing and energy.

- Take adrenal support supplements in the early afternoon to help sustain your energy to the evening.

- Stand up and stretch no matter where you are every hour.

So, now that you have some guidelines on how to build up a chronic case of fatigue as well as some ways to prevent and fix it, I encourage you to also ask yourself if your thought patterns, your stress level, or your general state of mind might be dragging and slowing you down. Take a good, long look at your lifestyle habits, like your food choices, eating patterns, sleep practices, exercise routines, and meditation practices, and make sure you have no leaks that energy could be draining out of. If you do the work consistently, in most cases your energy will be sustained. Just get to it.

Brilliant Energy Success Story: The High-Octane Superwoman

Brittany was a gem. She was one of the most impressive women I had ever met. She excelled in nearly everything she put her mind to. She worked like a dog and was intentional in every aspect of her health, life, and family. She used every single cell in her body for good. She maximized her talents as no one I had ever met. She was truly a remarkable person, mostly because she simply wanted to make a difference in the world, and clearly, she was.

Nine months prior to seeing me, Brittany had started a vegan diet. She had done quite a bit of reading about the benefits of a vegan lifestyle and wanted to give it a try. When she came to see me, she told me she had recently become plagued with headaches, dizziness, fatigue, and was completely hitting a wall in the afternoons. She normally liked to exercise first thing in the morning but found herself not able to get out of bed to hit the gym. She was noticing weight gain around her midsection and poor mood, with bouts of flying off the handle, wicked PMS, and tender breasts that she had not had in the past. Because her diet had always been so good, she had never supplemented with nutrients, and after talking to her for some time and then suggesting the needed tests, it became apparent that her diet may be the culprit.

Brittany's unfortunate mistake was that she had exchanged a complete protein diet with a severely protein deficient diet (not mixing enough vegetarian proteins to get the necessary amino acids and nutrients needed to feel balanced, energetic, and emotionally well). Additionally, she had started eating more sugar in her diet, due to intense cravings that were new to her. These things added up to a perfect dietary storm. The higher sugar diet had depleted her magnesium levels, her low-protein diet had left her deficient on amino acids that were causing her low-lying depression, and the higher intake of carbohydrates was causing her to have more cravings and fat gain.

Brittany's game plan included the following:

- Add more protein to her diet, eating along the Mediterranean style (low glycemic)

- Start intermittent fasting with meals between 10 a.m. and 7 p.m. only

- Weekly injections of B complex and glutathione, mood/PMS supplements, and DIM (diindolylmethane)

- Supplement with vitamin D, amino acids, vitamin C, and magnesium

- Optimize thyroid levels with medication, and correct the estrogen dominance with her female hormones

- Build in time for rest and recovery daily, with ten-minute power naps or silent times with no sensory input

These simple lifestyle changes and noninvasive treatments made a world of difference for Brittany, who was back to her old, truly remarkable self in record time. She lost belly fat quickly and was able to completely rid herself of the afternoon slump and dizziness, while her mood improved dramatically and she woke up daily feeling more rested. She has fewer mood swings and cravings for sugar and noticed that she went through an entire winter without getting sick. Her PMS resolved completely with progesterone treatment and supplementation

Treating women that have fatigue and exhaustion always makes me realize that there are so many effective ways to optimize your energy. What worked for Brittany may not be the right path for you, but that doesn't mean there is no path to overcoming your fatigue. Please do not accept the poor medical advice that "it is normal to feel zapped." Try to identify what might be dragging you down, and work to immediately eliminate it. Push for someone to help you optimize your health and hormones. As long as *you* work, *it* works!

10

Girls Squad: Why Fun and Friends Are *Vital* for Stress Control and Balance

"Friendship between women is different than friendship between men... It's my women friends that keep starch in my spine, and without them, I don't know where I would be."

—**JANE FONDA**

Having fun is an important part of everyone's life. And part of that entails spending quality time with others. Take the following quiz to see how you are doing in the fun department.

QUIZ: ARE YOU SOCIALLY ISOLATED?

1. Do you prefer emails or texts to face-to-face meetings? Y/N
2. Do you prefer staying in to going out on the weekends? Y/N

3. Does talking on the phone bother you? Y/N

4. Do you visit your family less than you used to? Y/N

5. Are you struggling with finding motivation? Y/N

6. When you are with your friends or family, do you find your mind wandering, thinking about what else you could be doing? Y/N

7. Are you more socially isolated than you were five years ago? Y/N

8. Do you find yourself spending most of your time catching up with friends and family via social media? Y/N

9. Does most of your communication with coworkers occur electronically? Y/N

10. Do you often find yourself too tired to want to socialize? Y/N

11. Do you belly laugh less than you used to? Y/N

12. Do your friends or family members exhaust you? Y/N

13. Do your friends joke about you never wanting to meet up or have fun? Y/N

14. Does your family insist that you are a workaholic? Y/N

If you answered yes to more than five of these questions, it's time to turn off your computer and your phone and head to your best friend's house, STAT! You are suffering from a lack of laughter, fun, and friendship. Basically, you're in danger of forgetting all the things that make life worth living. So let's fix it.

....

HOW DO SOCIAL CONNECTIONS IMPACT OUR STRESSFUL LIVES?

It's pretty clear that eating a healthy diet, exercising, taking the right supplements, sleeping deeply, meditating, and having balanced hormones are all factors vital for sustaining your brilliant self, long term. But another powerful strategy for maintaining your optimal health—and the one that is perhaps the most ignored—is by nourishing your connections with loved ones. However, in this new digital world we live in, doing this is deceptively difficult.

These days, we are all intricately connected to our friends and family through electronics—social media, email, and smart phones. We have more access to what is going on in these people's lives now more than ever. So, why are we still so socially disconnected? Why do people feel so alone?

Thirty years ago, when we were significantly less connected socially and technically, people relied on meeting up and talking in person over lunch, drinks, coffee, or on the phone. We didn't substitute an email for a face-to-face meeting. We didn't typically have more than 100 friends on a website where we posted three to four vapid sentences about what we are doing that moment (curse you, Zuckerberg!). We typically either kept that information to ourselves (as it probably should be) or saved it for when we got together with friends. Let's face it: We are sifting through a *lot* of communication and information from thousands of people every day. Humans are social beings. We're simply built that way, and we actually do live and survive through our social connections. That's why it's important to make sure those connections are real and meaningful and not simply words on a screen. The wonderful power of social behavior, or face-to-face encounters, can give us energy, heal many of our hurts, help to identify our weaknesses, bring out the best in us, and ultimately give us purpose.

Researchers at Brigham Young University looked at 148 studies on social interactions. They concluded that those who had planned, regular social interactions—including with family, friends, and colleagues—improved their long-term odds of survival by more than 50 percent. Surprisingly, those in the study who had limited or *no* social connectedness had a comparable heath status to someone who was smoking 15 cigarettes per day, drinking excessive amounts of alcohol, not exercising, or suffering from obesity.[35]

---

35 Julianne Holt-Lunstad, Timothy B. Smith, and J. Bradley Layton, "Social Relationships and Mortality Risk: A Meta-Analytic Review," *PLOS* (2010), doi:10.1371/journal.pmed.1000316.

And not only our physical health benefits from these encounters. Researcher Kenneth Kendler noted that social support through physical engagements with others reduced depression significantly in men and women.[36] Other research has shown that social connectedness supports the delicate stress response in the brain, providing significantly more controlled cortisol (stress hormone) production, which helps with anxiety, mood swings, glucose regulation, and sleep—all which ultimately affect our moods greatly. So let's stop hurting ourselves and start having a little fun. Keep reading for some quick tips that will help you make a face-to-face connection this week.

NO TIME FOR SOCIAL CONNECTIONS

Life's too short to waste in an endless mire of anxiety that comes from being overworked. It is a shame we have to grow up at all, because so many of the things we did as kids were so correct. As children, we were not overshadowed by worries, money problems, responsibilities, and constantly overthinking everything. Having fun was instinctual—stomping in puddles, lying around laughing, playing in the pool, riding bikes, and forming intense, connected friendships. We seem to lose this carefree attitude as we age, replacing it with deadlines, overcommitted schedules, stress-induced paralysis, and exhaustion to the point that we start saying no to everything fun.

And the irony is our demands—some material, others out of our control—hold us captive to a happiness that is forever elusive. Instead, in our endless quest, we become governed by feelings of exhaustion and inadequacy. We need to reclaim that sense of impulsive pleasure that went hand in hand with childhood.

36   Kenneth S. Kendler, "Classification of Psychopathology: Conceptual and Historical Background," *World Psychiatry: Official Journal of the World Psychiatric Association* 17, no. 3 (2018) 241-242, doi: 10.1002/wps.20549.

Life is full of moments of beauty, kindness, and triumph that we usually fail to notice because we're so wrapped up in our own concerns. Today we are inundated with messages like "Think big," "Go for more," and "Climb the ladder of success." But, if you are trying to do this without the help and support of others, it will be an unpleasant and lonely grind. And be selective—keep the people that you can laugh with the closest.

HOW LAUGHTER SUPPORTS STRESS RELIEF

As busy, highly stressed women, we tend to dismiss all forms of play. But psychologists have found that play—being silly, losing yourself in the moment, and engaging in something pointless but pleasurable—is essential to healthy relationships, stress reduction, and maintaining a sense of well-being. Laughing is one of the most positive, healthy, and easy things we can do for ourselves because it provides us with a huge lift, physically and emotionally. Plus, it's totally free.

Laughter reduces the levels of stress hormones, like cortisol and epinephrine (adrenaline), while also increasing the level of health-enhancing hormones, like endorphins. Laughter even increases the number of antibody-producing cells we have working for our immune system and enhances the overall effectiveness of T cells. All this means a stronger immune system and fewer manifestations of the physical effects of stress, like exhaustion, depression, insomnia, and weight gain.

When you engage in laughing, you experience a physical cleansing effect as well as a sort of emotional release. You also get a bit of a physical workout (assuming it's a good, belly laugh) from engaging the diaphragm, contracting the abdominal muscles, and stretching the shoulder muscles, leaving you more balanced and relaxed. Laughing is also great for the heart and increases oxygen levels throughout the body. The sad news, though, is that despite the enormous benefits of laughter, we are often just too tired, and we rarely take the time to indulge in a good belly laugh. Today, women do not laugh as we used to. Research suggests that healthy children may laugh as much as 400 times per day, but adults tend to laugh only 15 times per day, or sometimes not at all.[37] How depressing is that? Certainly that statistic is not a laughing matter. (I'm sorry. I couldn't help myself!)

Research shows that face-to-face communication and human connectedness have diminished in near direct correlation to the recent widespread use of electronic communication replacing direct, one-on-one communication.[38] This means we have been left with less communication, networking, touching, laughing, connection, and overall support from others. Other research has shown that the health benefits of laughter are even more far ranging than we ever before believed, showing that laughter can help relieve pain, bring greater happiness, and increase immunity.[39] Positive psychology even names the propensity for laughter and a sense of humor as one of the 24 signature strengths a person can possess.

SURROUND YOURSELF WITH OTHERS WHO LAUGH

Laughter connects us with others. It's as simple as that. The same as smiling and kindness (or even yawning), most people find that laughter is irresistibly contagious. Therefore, if you laugh more, you can most likely help others around you to laugh more, and they will be happier as well. By elevating the mood of those around you, you can reduce their stress levels

---

37 Rod A. Martin and Nicholas A. Kuiper, "Daily Occurrence of Laughter: Relationships with Age, Gender, and Type A Personality," *International Journal of Humor Research* 12, no. 4 (1999): 355–384, doi: 10.1515/humr.1999.12.4.355.

38 Emily Drago, "The Effect of Technology on Face-to-Face Communication," *Elon Journal of Undergraduate Research in Communications* 6, no. 1 (2015): 13–19.

39 Mary Payne Bennett and Cecile Annette Lengacher, "Humor and Laughter May Influence Health: III. Laughter and Health Outcomes," *Evidence-Based Complementary and Alternative Medicine* 5, no. 1 (2007): 37–40, doi: 10.1093/ecam/nem041.

as well as yours and perhaps improve the quality of social interactions you experience with them, reducing everyone's stress level even more.

Have you ever caught a case of the giggles with someone else at an inappropriate time even though you knew you shouldn't be laughing? And then, by the time you manage to stop, the situation somehow doesn't seem so bad anymore? I have—at a funeral! The point is, though, that I truly love the fact that laughter softens difficult moments. I have thankfully surrounded myself with funny friends who continuously bring joy to my life and make the bad moments seem a little more bearable. Nearly every friend of mine is funny and loves to make me laugh. Laughing, smiling, and enjoying one another is truly one of the best ways to diminish a tough, stressful, or negative situation. Laughter brings the focus away from anger, negativity, hopelessness, bitterness, and guilt like nothing else can. Humor gives us a lighter perspective and can even help us change our view of certain situations so that something that seemed threatening can become simply a minor obstacle.

Above all, laughter and playful behavior offer a sense of engagement. The act of laughing can bring you into the moment, which is something desperately needed by highly stressed women who are on rigid schedules in their day and are often always thinking about the next thing that needs to get done. The act of play and laughter are one of the few aspects of our lives that are not about the outcome but the acts themselves, and that is so healing. The joy in work is often lost because we are all so serious, trying to muddle through our busy day. When we lack episodes of laughter, connections, and touch, we easily begin to feel that our daily duties are laborious, painful, and downright frustrating. We have unfortunately lost our playfulness and silliness, only to exchange them over time with deadlines, dread, and exhaustion. And in doing this, we have also surrounded ourselves with those who are like the people we have become: serious workaholics who are no fun at all.

BALANCING YOUR FRIENDSHIPS

I have told women countless times in my lectures that in order to have less stress, more room for creativity, and less angst, they need to group all of their connections (aka, any people they come into regular contact with: family, friends, coworkers, neighbors, etc.) into three categories: energizers, neutralizers, and drainers. I am always amazed at how successful, dynamic women notoriously surround themselves with others who drain the life out of them. However, this is something that can be easily avoided if you take more care to recognize the types of people in your life. It is a simple task to put your contacts into three categories, and I would strongly suggest that you do so as soon as possible.

Energizers

These people make you feel light, happy, energetic, and positive. They support you and lift you up even if you are only in their presence for a matter of minutes. This is the type of person who should always be your best friend.

Neutralizers

These people do not make you feel up or down. They do not change how you feel when you are with them. They are totally neutral. You can take them or leave them, and typically they do not elicit any emotional response from you when they are around. These are people like your dry cleaner, mailman, or the distant cousin you only talk to at family reunions. You know, boring people.

Drainers

After you are with a drainer, you will likely either need to load up on sugar, drain a bottle of wine, scream into a pillow, stress eat some french fries, or take a nap. These kinds of people take you down like a two-ton anchor. Everyone knows someone like this, and you probably have someone specific in mind. They make you feel helpless, angry, frustrated, used, and exhausted. Worst of all, they typically never change, and they will suck the life out of you when given even the slightest opportunity. The real reason you need to worry about these kinds of people, though, is because they are also attracted to success and women who have their sh** together. So be aware. These are toxic people, and having you continue to feed into their drama will likely only perpetuate the situation. It's time to say good-bye to drainers and stack the deck with energizers.

GOING WITH THE FLOW

Think about a moment when you were really in the zone, a time when you were crushing a work presentation you had down pat, enjoying an especially good yoga session, or recounting your favorite anecdote to a group of cackling friends. You probably felt amazing, almost invincible, in that moment. Wouldn't it be great if you could experience more of that feeling? Psychologist Mihaly Csikszentmihalyi coined the term *flow* to explain a peak moment of consciousness when we are so engaged in what we are doing that we lose all sense of time amid a state of deep enjoyment and satisfaction. Sounds pretty great on paper, and in practice it is even better. The problem is that we have too few of these experiences when we are so busy and have no time for fun.

While I have not personally mastered this flow by any stretch of the imagination, it is a key component for women's stress management. Unfortunately, most brilliant women do not do this naturally. We are planners, doers, and surveyors—plotting our attacks every day. We don't hang back and go with the flow. We are focused on output, delivering, and getting it all done.

But we are not machines. If you are constantly worrying about what comes next and never letting yourself go with the flow, it may well be time for a life shift in this area. Again, don't be ashamed to admit you struggle here; this is a common problem for brilliant women. If we ever are in the flow, it's probably only for an hour on Saturday when we're too exhausted to do otherwise. Here are some questions you need to ask yourself when you find yourself saying, "I have no time to relax and go with the flow."

- Is there anything I can say no to that would open up more time for flow and doing things like meeting friends, sitting and reading, or taking a short vacation?

- Will what I am doing matter in one week, one month, or one year? Is it important enough that I can't take a break from it to do something refreshing and fun?

- Do I make myself a priority? Am I so busy being professional and meeting goals that I'm neglecting personal growth and self-care?

- Do I accept where I am in my own personal journey? Are my expectations of what I need to accomplish reasonable? Should I step back and reevaluate my direction and then make changes to build in more playtime while still achieving my career and professional goals?

- Do I leave myself enough days off? Are there days in the month that have nothing on the calendar—purposely?

- When is the last time I changed my routine, took a different route to work, made it a priority to be with friends regularly, stopped off at a family member's home spontaneously, or unexpectedly took the kids to the beach instead of school for the day?

Once you answer these questions, set yourself a goal, give yourself a clear space of time without any interruptions to achieve it in, and focus on the enjoyment of the process of being in the flow to enhance self-esteem, confidence, happiness, and overall satisfaction. What could be better than that?

LIVE IN THE PRESENT—DON'T OVERTHINK IT

The reality is that brilliant women are overthinkers. This is one of the fundamental reasons for our success. We think and we do. But as time marches on, this virtue can turn against us, and we often develop a strong tendency to overthink things and worry about things that either have happened, haven't happened, could happen, or might happen.

Needless to say, this worrying is not good for us. With our busy lives and never-ending to-do lists, most women end up looking back at some point and realizing that all of the worry, regret, overthinking, and painful blow-ups—most of which were completely unnecessary—robbed them of joy. Joy that was often right in front of them if they had just taken a moment to live in the present instead of obsessing over what could be. So, while our brilliant minds are the key to our excellence, they can also often work as our enemy.

We also worry too much about our pasts. The constant replaying of unwanted memories, painful experiences, lost time, and the inability to get a perspective on things is one of the biggest things holding us back. A long while ago, I read that if you are feeling regretful, sad, frustrated, or angry, that the only thing keeping you stuck in these agonizing feelings is that you keep *thinking* about them. Overthinking prevents you from enjoying the present. You ignore the here and now—the person next to you, the meeting you should be listening to, or how beautiful the world is, while you are consumed by your thoughts of something that happened in the past. And this effect only gets worse the longer you dwell on them. Overthinking leads to anxiety, frustration, anger, indecision, and self-doubt, which we brilliant women simply have no time for.

STOP TRYING TO BE PERFECT

Logically, we know that perfection is a myth. It's something we have conjured up in our minds that doesn't actually exist, and yet that doesn't stop us striving for it. We hold ourselves up to impossible standards, trying to be funnier, younger looking, smarter, and fitter and with a flawless work ethic to boot. And while bettering yourself is a good thing, this process of chasing perfection is exhausting and unattainable.

Women in the workforce are trying to succeed in their careers while managing to dress well, exercise, diet, and use polite and friendly etiquette. Antiquated social constructs dictate that we have to try to look attractive, maintain a tidy living space, and act demure around our male counterparts. It takes enormous vigilance to maintain this façade of perfection on all fronts. It's the Stepford Wives image superimposed on the frame of Hillary Clinton. But really, it's our internal stress hormones getting the better of us.

This quest for perfection erodes our vital hormones and interrupts our sleep. Ultimately, it leads to depression, anxiety, and many other medical disorders. And it is a problem that affects women disproportionately to men. I see women in our offices more often than men with the common complaint of stress-induced emotional and physical problems. In fact, the rates of anxiety are 50 percent higher in women, often because they are manifesting physical symptoms of their inner turmoil from the societally induced disease of stress and perfection.[40] So banish perfection

---

40 Peta Slocombe, "Australia's Biggest Mental Health Check-in: Going from Talk to Action," *Newcastle Herald*, April 18, 2018, https://www.theherald.com.au/story/5348200/mental-health-going-from-talk-to-action/.

from your mind and life, and instead accept that the bad comes with the good. But most of all, remember that whatever you do is good enough.

As you continue to advance your career or business or parenting skills, please strive to let go of the tendency to be perfect. Try to take risks, love your body, and, most importantly, give yourself permission to make some mistakes once in a while. By giving yourself this license (which, frankly, is the least you can do), you free yourself up to try new things, which allows you to be more innovative, creative, and confident. Giving yourself permission to be less than perfect also builds on your leadership skills and even enables you to be a better problem-solver. Most importantly, however, it demonstrates to others that you're human, and when you're human, you're relatable. And when you're relatable, you're not only a good leader. You're a *great* leader—and a brilliant woman.

FAST TRACK: GETTING SOCIAL AND HAVING FUN

We all have responsibilities in our lives that cause us stress, sometimes even to the point that having fun feels like an unnecessary luxury. However, including fun activities in your life is one of the best remedies for stress relief. While many responsible adults have adult-sized responsibilities that make it easy to put fun on the low end of the priorities list, letting your inner child come out to play can keep you feeling vital and happy. Let's get you back to enjoying your life again. It's what makes it worth living.

- Don't use the internet as your *only* form of social interaction. This superficial connection is often not deep enough to really help some-one feel "heard," confirmed, supported, or energized. You need to have other social connections too, and should make it a priority to meet with people face-to-face. If you have no friends or family to confide in, find someone and be the best friend you can be for them. Give it time to grow and make sure you are giving of yourself to the relationship to help it mature.

- Visit or meet up with a neighbor, coworker, or relative that you do not typically spend much time with. Have you met someone you would like to get to know more? Now is your time. Make it a point to call them and see if you can make a deeper connection.

- Engage in a group sports activity or go on a walk with someone. Not only are walking and sports activities great for you physically, but they also are a wonderful way to break the ice, loosen you up, and connect to other people with something in common to talk about initially.

- Go on a date! This could be with your partner, or you can go on a double date with another couple. It could also be a date with someone new you've been wanting to get to know. It could be with anyone that you feel would enhance your connections.

- Socialize as a family. While this may seem like a thing of the past, families who take the time to meet with other families socially encourage connectedness and family bonding. Give it a try some time. Have your neighbors over for dinner and games.

- Get out from behind your TV or computer screen. Real relationships are largely nonverbal. You have to be face-to-face to communicate well and connect.

- Volunteer. Do something that helps others and has a beneficial effect on how you feel about yourself!

- Be a "joiner." Find groups that will help open you up to common interests and potential friends.

- Write to a family member. Tell them how much you appreciate them.

- Call a friend. Don't email them; call them! Ultimately this is about being in your friends' lives. Show up for those you love!

- Recognize the moments that work. Each day, pay attention to at least one or two moments when things fall into place and allow you to move through your day easier. This will help you stay on a positive track.

- Put down your work and call it a day. Enough said.

- Load up on funny friends. Find two or three funny friends who will for sure make you laugh from your belly.

- Host a potluck dinner party. You have to have dinner anyway, so why not invite some friends over? With everyone bringing a dish, it won't cost much, and it's a great opportunity to connect with friends.

- Invite your favorite people over for a comedy movie night. There is no better stress reliever than laughter, and laughing with your friends makes it even better.

- Reconnect with nature. A little sunlight, listening to the sounds of nature, breathing in the fresh air, and feeling the wind on your face are great, cost-free, and immediate ways to reduce stress that most people don't often think to do.

- Find humor in your life. Instead of complaining about life's frustrations, try to laugh about them. This may be difficult at first, but if something is so frustrating or depressing that it's ridiculous, realize that you will probably look back on it and laugh. It is likely you will find yourself being more lighthearted and silly with this approach to your problems (something we could all use more of).

- Fake it until you make it. Just as studies show the positive effects of smiling occur whether the smile is fake or real, faked laughter also provides the benefits mentioned earlier. The body can't distinguish between fake laughter and real laughter. The physical benefits are exactly the same, and the former usually leads to the latter anyway. So, smile more and fake laugh; you'll still achieve positive effects, and the fake merriment may lead to real smiles and laughter.

Brilliant Fun Success Story

Andy was a bit of an introvert but loved her job as a nurse. She worked hard and was promoted after a short period of time. But when she came to see me, she was convinced she would not be able to be in a leadership position mainly because she felt lacking in her communication skills and was not comfortable having face-to-face conversations. While she grew up highly socialized, she admitted that most of her communication was texting, social media, and emails (a situation I am sadly starting to see more and more of). She had few friends and considered her dogs to be the most supportive "people" in her life. This is sweet, but ultimately not very effective.

She avoided parties and holiday get-togethers and found that she felt better being alone, especially after working all week. Over time, this habit of being alone became more imbedded in her. She felt tired a great deal of the time and admitted that her enthusiasm for life was not what she wanted it to be. She found herself being more negative, petty, judgmental, and even raging at times. She wanted to know if her hormones were normal and what she might be able to do about this to excel in her new leadership position.

After testing and evaluation, it was apparent that the modern-day antisocial connectedness environment had stunted her ability to see the world or even communicate on a level that was comfortable for her. She had some minor hormone abnormalities, but they were the least of her worries. Nevertheless, together, Andy and I put together a plan that addressed her low testosterone and progesterone levels and her need for social connection to help her escape the isolation she had imposed on herself and get her feeling like the brilliant woman she really was.

HER GAME PLAN INCLUDED THE FOLLOWING:

- Immediately treating the low testosterone and progesterone levels she was experiencing in the luteal phase of her cycle

- Reaching out to old friends every week, setting meetings with them, and going out with them even when she didn't feel like it

- Spending more time engaging with her immediate family

- Taking classes in leadership and public speaking

- Engaging with other leaders at her hospital

- Calling at least three people every week just to talk

- Limiting her time on social media

- Beginning a journal to track how she was feeling and to list ways in which she could correct her unrealistic goals of perfection

But did it work? I've never seen this kind of mental transformation in a person before or since. In six months, Andy was nearly recovered from her fear of being a social misfit and was asked to give a lecture at work about social connectedness and how we can improve our mood, energy, and brain function by spending time with others, connecting with them, and being present. And I'm happy to report that she nailed her leadership role with flying colors.

11

The Brilliant Vibe Tribe: Creating Personal Support Systems with the *Right People* to Keep You Accountable, Supported, and Balanced

*"Surround yourself with the dreamers and the doers,
the believers and the thinkers, but most of all,
surround yourself with those who see the greatness
within you, even when you don't see it yourself."*
—*EDMUND LEE*

Being part of a tribe is important to feeling supported and nurtured in your everyday life. Take the following quiz to see how strong your existing tribe is.

QUIZ: DO YOU NEED TO WORK ON BUILDING YOUR TRIBE?

....

1. Do you feel as if you are supporting everyone around you and always have to be the strong one? Y/N

2. Do you feel that very few people would even understand the level of stress and pressure you are under? Y/N

3. Do you find yourself wishing you could enjoy the company of others but also know that there is just not enough time in the week to accomplish this? Y/N

4. Do you see yourself as a loner at times? Y/N

5. Are you jealous of those girl trips that everyone else seems to have time for? Y/N

6. Are you lacking close friends who will let you know when you are on the wrong path or about to make a bad decision? Y/N

7. Do you find yourself wanting a tribe who can support you, understand you, and help you develop your unique gifts? Y/N

8. Have you begun to feel that you are in desperate need of more laughter and less seriousness in your life? Y/N

9. Do you feel you have no one to talk to? Y/N

10. Do you feel as though there are few people that get you? Y/N

11. Are you relying solely on your significant other to be your everything? Y/N

If you answered yes to more than four of the above questions, then it is high time you start the serious hunt for your tribe. Don't put this off until another time when "things slow down." This is far too important to your life and sanity. The time for tribe building is now.

....

WHY A TRIBE?

I consider myself extremely lucky to be born into a supportive, loving family and to be blessed with more friends and amazing coworkers than I deserve. And I do not take these people for granted. Ever. But it wasn't always that way.

I have been on this earth for 54 years now, and I'm sad to say that I didn't take my friendships as seriously as I should have during the years I probably needed them the most. Now, of course, I know better. And the fact that I continue to meet remarkable men and women who may become part of my tribe on my journey through this life is one of the most welcoming surprises in my life. The happy fact is that incredible people keep showing up. You just have to be open to them.

Your tribe is the group of people you surround yourself with whom you know you can count on no matter what. I like to define the idea of a tribe like this: A tribe is a group of people who come together with common values and the desire to be present in one another's lives. A tribe is created over time. It is your chosen family of friends that choose to stand by you no matter what.

Tribes are essential for success and sanity when you are busy changing the world. This is because behind every brilliant woman are usually ten other brilliant women supporting her. But this support system doesn't magically appear, and it can take quite a while to construct. The process of making a tribe is something I feel is important to discuss for brilliant women because we often do not take the time or energy to even contemplate that it is necessary for the health of your heart, soul, and mind. To be clear, your tribe isn't simply helping you get work done; their role is much deeper than that. The fact that your tribe "sees you" is, in my opinion, the reason why you need them in your life. This is a concept that shows up in the movie *Avatar*. (I *love* that movie.) And I think the reason I love it so much and have watched it so many times is that the Na'vi (the proper name for the alien race in the movie) could see each other on a deep, emotional level and would tell each other this. And I think that having a tribe or significant other that "sees you" in this way is one of the most vital ingredients for your ongoing successes.

Are there people in your life who truly see you? Do you have a few people who will help you stay on the right path, will love you no matter what, and will be there for you when you can't take one more step? Do you have people who have your back, will provide for you when you can't, will prop you up, will defend you, go to bat for you, or cry with you when you need it? Do you have someone you can call at the last moment to go out and just laugh with? You should. You need a tribe that "sees you" exactly as you are so when you can't see yourself, they can help you find your way. The value of a tribe for a brilliant woman is in providing a sense of nurturing that is vital to their success. Unfortunately, asking for this nurturing does not come natural to brilliant women because we are too busy nurturing others. But this type of help is instrumental for the personal and spiritual growth of successful women.

A tribe can help you with new ideas and a network. They can reel you back in when you get way out on a limb, support you when you feel you are at the end of your rope, and ultimately remind you who you are. Most importantly, a good tribe will not judge you but help you be the best version of yourself. There is a deep sense of safety that comes with having people you are deeply connected to and can trust. And as much as we like to think of ourselves as invincible, we need a tribe we can rely on.

Here are some of the rewards you'll reap for your efforts in building a tribe:

- Support when you feel like giving up
- More energy and strength than you could ever generate alone

- Enrichment through many lifelong relationships

- An encouraging community that allows you to make your passion your livelihood

- Feeling like the luckiest woman in the world to be surrounded by those who care about you and have your back

- And perhaps the greatest—and most unexpected—gift is that leading a community will serve as a catalyst for you to become a better human being

How to Create a Tribe

So now that you know why you need a tribe, how do you create one? Well, that's easier said than done. Successful women are often loners and don't gravitate to those who truly see them, let alone understand or support them. This is a problem, as it creates sadness, loneliness, resentment, and distrust and usually leads to retreating further into work. So, step one in building a tribe is to let more people into your life. How? Often this is as simple as asking them.

Since I started earnestly asking for those people in my life that I can be real with—those who make me laugh, keep my secrets, listen to me, support me, guide me, and hold me accountable—the most amazing group of people has shown up, several of which were there all along. As soon as I started letting these people into my life, things began shifting for me. I started to more fully come into myself, my business took off more than expected, and I was able to have more fun. The tribe you develop will show you parts of yourself that you didn't know existed. They will show you things about yourself that you forgot were there, and they will help you be even braver than you already are.

The creation of a tribe is a process and needs to be a priority for any brilliant woman who wants to be sane and happy long term. Let's get into some tips on how to find your tribal support group. The following are some steps you can take to build your tribe:

- Be mindful and set your intentions on what you want to find. Put it out there. Ask for friends, a soul mate, or for your tribe to show up for you. Ask for the things you need (e.g., laughing more, trusting more, being supported more, listened to more, or having someone to spark creativity). In other words, ask for exactly what you need to feel supported and healthy.

- Take the time to be with others. Your tribe will most likely be made up, partially, by those who are in your life now, but you are not taking the time to connect with them. This is why you must create experiences where you can get to know them and they you. This might mean putting something on your calendar weekly or monthly where you spend time with them and can be in a situation where you are not distracted or stressed out. Ideally, this will end up being something you want to do, so have fun with it!

- Be discerning, but not full of judgment. Your tribe will most likely consist of others who are like you in many ways and yet are the complete opposite in others. Your tribe might be partially made up of those different enough from you that they will be laid back, spontaneous, not scheduled, and will make you laugh till you pee in your pants. These tribal members can sometimes have bad habits that conflict with how you usually live your life, but they will keep you balanced more than you can imagine—and they are a hell of a lot of fun, too. They will keep you understanding the importance of spontaneity and remind you that the little things in life are still worth paying. That said, bad habits and inconsistency can rub off, and you should always be sure that these relationships are building you up, not dragging you down. So be discerning to make sure they bring out the best in you, and set boundaries to ensure that you can keep your heart open but not be taken advantage of.

- Surround yourself with like-minded people. Find a community of people who feel authentic. Find those who share the same beliefs, are creative, and are excited about life as you are. Look for people who want to make the world a better place and are motivated like you. In the right environment, both parties will benefit. So, reach out to people and show them who you are. Make sure they understand you, or at least want to understand you and are not aiming to control you. That type of dynamic simply will not work. Ultimately, we cannot feel at home with people who do not understand who we are as people. So, make sure seeking out like-minded souls is a big component of your tribe-building process.

- Find activities that you can engage in to meet others. Sign up for an art class, women's group, or a spiritual retreat. Take time for a trip to learn something new like surfing or meditation or whatever sounds good. Then, talk to others about it and invite them to come along. Your next best friend could be in the same class, if you keep your eyes open for them.

- Listen to how you feel when you meet new people. How do you feel when you meet them or get to know them? Do you feel you have known them your whole life? Do you feel excited when you are with them? How does the conversation feel? You want to find those who make you light up. Stop looking at your phone and thinking of what you have to get done that day. Instead, listen to yourself and how you feel. Take action and be brave enough to invite them to something you are doing or to lunch, drinks, or coffee. Get to know them. Make time for this, and I promise you it will pay off.

Consider starting to blog about this. Or, better yet, start a women's group and invite a few people who are like minded and then see where it goes from there. Trust the process.

You are unique, not weird. Sometimes our quest to find those who can understand us is undermined by the fact that we believe we are different and that no one will understand us. We spend most of our life fixing everyone else, and then we never see how *we* need to be fixed. While you may be unique or different, if you build your tribe well, they will be more like you than you think. Especially if they know who they are and can see you as you can see them. No masks, no ego. If you can keep these principles in mind, you should have no trouble building a strong, supportive tribe in no time.

We can get so wrapped up in our busy lives that we don't take time to nurture ourselves or build meaningful relationships. As the internet and social media become a larger part of our day, we forget about the fruitful exchanges we can have with individuals. The ultimate benefit of having a group of soul sisters boils down to the fact that we as humans are social beings who are spending more and more time isolating ourselves in our crazy busy lives. Add on top of this, there is so much tearing down of women in society, and much of this comes from other women when we should uplift each other. We have the power to change the conversation when women are being torn down about their bodies, their choices, about how they present themselves to the world—and instead lead by example by having healthy, happy female friendships.

WHY BRILLIANT WOMEN ISOLATE THEMSELVES

For years, I have counseled women who isolate themselves. Every week, I see women hull themselves up in their work and choose not to be supported by their husbands, friends, or family. Brilliant women are notorious for this. They are so capable and achievement oriented in every area of their life that the people in their lives tend to stay out of their way. Sometimes, they even convince themselves that it's better this way, but I am here to assure you that it is not. Women often isolate themselves for several reasons:

- They prefer not to be honest about how they are feeling, as it makes them look not so brilliant.

- They would rather throw themselves into their work because it gives them something they can't get anywhere else.

- They have been burned too many times by someone and can't seem to find those who will love and accept them unconditionally without adding more drama to their lives.

- They have learned to shut down who they really are—to protect themselves from rejection—while their true selves become hidden from themselves and others.

The difficult pill to swallow here is that the more successful we are and the harder we work, the more imbalanced our lives become—unless we have a tribe who surrounds us, keeping us accountable in every life area. This, in particular, is something I have struggled with most of my life. It is probably one of the reasons I have been so addicted to work. But about ten years ago I realized that I was majorly missing out on the support and love that others so want to give, and I had no idea at the time I needed it so badly.

THE BENEFITS OF BEING PART OF A TRIBE

I have since learned having a supportive tribe is not only beneficial, it is essential to a brilliant woman's success. Some things that a good tribe can bring to the table are laughter, honesty, clarity, listening, direction, advice, and support. Having a tribe also affects you positively in the following ways:

- It reduces stress. Let's face it, if you've had a hell of a day—one you spent dodging bullets and having things literally fall apart all around you—a trip out with friends nearly always snaps you out of it. Bonding is a biological response for women that soothes the nerves and reduces the stress response.

- It creates accountability. We need to have women (and sometimes men) who keep us accountable to ourselves to share our goals and dreams with. I still remember when one of my closest friends called me after I made the decision to open a new business (which I had no time for) and asked if she could order a psychiatric consultation for me. While we may not always listen to the advice from our tribe, at the very least, it does cause us to pause and know we are being held accountable when we need it.

- It provides you with the cold, hard truth. Hearing the truth can be tricky for strong women (usually because the truth is that you often scare others), but you will need at least one member of your tribe who is able to tell you the cold, hard truth, no matter what. They need to be able to point out when you are screwing up. We are all human, and this is bound to happen with all you have going on, but in the midst of chaos, you often cannot see things objectively. Having an honest person who loves you point this out is beyond priceless. However, it is imperative that they not only point these things out but are also there for you to give you suggestions on how to get back on track or slow it down a bit. Otherwise, they aren't a friend; they're a critic.

- It allows you to nurture and be nurtured. This is part of our DNA as women. We are driven to nurture others, but we are also more receptive to and healed by nurturing that comes our way. This is something that is non-negotiable for us. We have to have nurturing in our lives, both giving and receiving. You will be happier, nicer, and much more complete if you can continue to take care of others while letting your guard down so others can take care of you, too. When you support others and let them support you, it is not only rewarding but also allows you to stay strong and with an open heart.

- It provides you with soul mates. Along my path I have found many soul mates—women and men you share something with on such a deep level that you don't even understand it. Often, you know it within the first five minutes of meeting them. It may feel as if you've known them for some time, even though you just met. These precious humans make up the inner circle of your tribe. The key here is to understand that no *one* person will be everything to you, which is why you need a tribe!

- You will have optimal support. This community of women (and men) can help support your goals and objectives and keep you lifted up when you feel as though you are drowning. Surround yourself with people who have vision, courage, love, and spirituality and are continually achieving personal development. They will keep you inspired and motivated to do the same.

BRILLIANT WOMEN NEED SUPPORTIVE PARTNERS

I know it can be hard to talk about, but this is a topic that I feel must be addressed, because it seems to be more common than not with brilliant women. Women who have success and are achievement oriented often find themselves feeling alone, unsupported, and unmatched with their mates. They find themselves pulling most of the weight and are more often than not the breadwinners in their family. And this leads to feelings of resentment.

Women who make things happen in this world are often attracted to easygoing, lighthearted, laid-back partners. You know the ones: they make you laugh and they're the life of the party. They don't take things too seriously. This is exactly the kind of guy overachieving women are attracted to, because we all wish we had a bit more of that easiness in ourselves.

But over time, a pattern usually reveals itself. The busier person in the relationship gets the most done and takes on the most responsibilities, simply because they can. Women and their partners begin with what appears to be the perfect ebb and flow. But this doesn't last. Inevitably, what ends up happening—because we all like things done a certain way—is that for some insane reason we brilliant women keep piling on more and more of the other's responsibilities onto us because we can do it faster, better, and without having to be reminded a hundred times. This entire scenario, with around a decade of gradual development, creates a giant mess.

The brilliant woman then becomes frustrated and more exhausted because she now has to deal with the house, the kids, the car, and the finances while her partner takes fewer and fewer of the responsibilities over time. Inevitably, resentment kicks in, and the brilliant woman begins to not like her life so much. I have found that while partners have good intentions and want to be there for their high-achieving, breadwinning significant others, the reality in their minds is that it's just easier for the super accomplished brilliant woman to take care of everything, because she is good at it and likes it done a certain way.

Emotional Stalemate

So, what happens when brilliant women find themselves at an emotional stalemate with their partner? They feel something is lacking in their relationship and that they are getting taken advantage of, but it happened so gradually that they're not able to fully explain how they feel or ultimately deal with the mounting resentment, disappointment, and fear that they might not be able to keep up with the growing list of responsibilities. It doesn't help that the majority of male partners are often unable to meet the emotional day-to-day needs of the women they are with, and this gets progressively worse as time goes on. When a relationship starts, we don't yet have as much going on in our lives. Business success, having kids, and trying to juggle daily chores in the midst of it all come later. And the easygoing personality of the mate you used to love soon becomes annoying.

The truth is, though, that it's not all our partner's fault. You both had a role to play in creating this situation. Mates (and I really mean men here) are often at a loss because they *want* to help but find themselves pushed to the sidelines every time, so it's just easier for most to stay there and out of your way. In fact, they think it's what we want them to do. Brilliant women find themselves no longer being able to open up to their partners, because we aren't able to give them what they need. We often suffer silently and feel as if we are not being heard or seen and, in time, close off to our partners. This is a vicious cycle that usually does not end well unless one or both partners are willing to step in to make drastic changes and stick with them.

What Brilliant Women Need from Their Partners

Brilliant women are powerhouses. However, to be at our best, we also need the following from our partners, because let's face it, we can't (and shouldn't) do it all alone:

- To feel loved

- To feel safe

- To feel supported

- To be nurtured

- To be appreciated

- To be desired

- To feel our partner can be counted on

Strong women still need their partners to be strong, create a safe environment, and have their back. They need to know that when the chips are down and they can't go on that their partner has things under control. And above all, they need to be able to depend on them to be strong and emotionally supportive. Women must have these things to keep on the brilliant path—to keep the momentum, knowing that the one person she adores the most is right there with her every step of the way.

Women need their partners to *care* enough to take the time to listen, pay attention, and support them when they need it. They often give the impression that they are fine all by themselves and don't need anybody's help. However, this is one of the biggest untruths about brilliant women. In fact, brilliant women may need their partners and their tribe more than anyone else. Women who are independent can easily understand a man or mate who is also independent and career driven and respect when they have life goals. But successful, independent women do not need or want their mate to define who they are as a person. They want someone who is willing to support them and be by their side, but not to own them. They are not dependent on their partners, because they have a life of their own and are too busy creating a living on their own terms.

Brilliant, high-achieving women have developed habits of discipline and hard work that spill over into their relationships, making them extremely devoted to keeping the relationship alive. These women are committed, dedicated, and loyal beyond belief, but they are also likely to be decisive and will not put up with something that is not fair or support-ive. Unfortunately, even when everything else is going well, it is all too common for a mate to be intimidated by a woman more successful than them, which is likely to cause relationship problems. Communicating with your partner and making them a more integral, purpose-filled part of your tribe can help with this, but in the end the outcome is depen-dent primarily on your partner's strength of character. So, what character traits should highly successful women hope to find in a partner?

Strong Partnerships

Above all, brilliant women are seeking relationships that are a two-way street: they want to know that their partners have their game together and are plugged in, secure, and strong. This is because a person who is comfortable with a driven and ambitious woman will likely need to be on a similar path or, at minimum, engaged fully in life to understand and appreciate the hustle we take part in. Any partner who needs reassurance and validation from a woman who is strong and independent will likely not find it in the long term. A brilliant woman expects her mate to be self-assured and self-reliant, and while she will easily support and care for them, she typically will not find it acceptable to have to continually prop them up and remind them how much she needs them—because she doesn't. This is sometimes a controversial idea, and it brings up all sorts of interesting talking points, but I feel it is important to discuss, because I hear this over and over in my office.

Strong women do not tolerate a mate who cannot stand on his own, and over time a relationship like this will not work. We all need love and affection and to share gratitude for each other; those things cannot be overlooked. But the unique dynamics of a brilliant woman's needs in a relationship cannot be disregarded, either.

A strong man will not expect to be needed by a woman of this caliber, but it is important to note that men still want to feel wanted, and we all still need love and affection to feel valued in a relationship. Brilliant women also need their mates to take the reins at times. Just because they are in a leadership position or in charge during the day does not mean that they need to shoulder the same in the responsibilities at home or with children. At the end of the day, a strong woman still appreciates a partner who makes plans, romances her, takes the lead sometimes, and treats her like a princess. While brilliant women often like to be in control, they still very much desire their mates to step up at times, and this should be something that is discussed between them to set up mutual boundaries and expectations. Most importantly, the support of a mate for a brilliant woman must be unwavering. Strong women need to feel secure in the fact that they will not be betrayed or lose support from their partners, especially when things get tough.

To put all of this as simply as I can: The right man for a strong woman is one who knows to stand in front of her when she needs protection, behind her when she needs support, and beside her when she needs a partner. I know that may sound corny. But it's the truth. And coming to terms with this idea, as well as clearly defining you and your partner's specific relationship needs, is a fundamental part of forming a strong and supportive tribe.

FAST TRACK TO A BRILLIANT TRIBE

Congratulations! Whether you read the entire chapter—taking notes in the margins and vision-boarding the main ideas—or just skipped to this section for the quick tips, I'm glad you made it. So, here is a condensed list of ways to create a tribe of your own that will help you build a fuller, happier, and more engaging brilliant life.

- Start with a clear intention and a desire to have the tribe you want. Consider listening to women or men talk, and see how you feel in their presence. For example, do you feel supported, enlightened, or engaged? Can you see this person standing strong for you? Find common threads in those women out there whom you feel you can share things with to help you find more people who might be able to relate to you.

- Start small and stay focused. You don't need to get ten women in your group by week one. Pace yourself, and don't feel obligated to bring a member into your tribe that you know will be more work than you the have time or energy for. This is your tribe. Treat it like a think tank—a support group of women who share similar goals, attitudes, or philosophies, working to create something none of them could create alone. Think of the qualities you want your tribe to have. For instance, start with merits like doesn't judge, has a sense of humor, is an artist, lives with wide-open passion, and is loyal. Look especially for one or two potential tribe members who don't freak out about the small stuff, as this is important to have in a highly stressed woman's tribe.

- Take an inventory of your current friends and family. This will help you determine if you already have the start of a tribe right in front of you. Stay true to what you want in your inner circle. Remember, you shouldn't feel obligated to include someone just because you have known them your whole life.

- Listen to your inner voice and instincts. Listen to your gut feeling about a person. Your body will tell you. Do you feel drawn to them right away, as though you've known them for years? Or do they make you put up your guard? Make good choices and listen to yourself. You don't need any more drama.

- Pay attention to their social media posts. This is a great way to root out the crazies. Do you like what you see? Is it for real? Consider starting a blog on something of interest—dogs, cooking, artwork, hiking, etc.—and see if like-minded people show up in the comments.

- Consider doing something you are passionate about (besides working): go to a class, join a club, or learn something new that you have always been interested in. Doing this might lead you to others with similar interests.

- Begin spending time with these women. Ask them if they want to meet for coffee or a glass of wine before going home or to go on a Saturday hike. Get to know them, and then make up your mind if this person has the qualities to be in your inner circle.

- Consider being deliberate about finding your tribe. Find two women you adore and trust and ask them to find two other women they adore. Sometimes women brought in by other women are the best tribal members you can find, and you may not have found them unless your friend introduced them to you first.

- Find a common interest between you and your potential tribe members, and invite them over. This could be a book club, hiking group, entrepreneurial group, retreat, and so on. Try to stay off your phone and instead open up your heart and talk to others in the group and see how it feels. Keep it purposeful.

- Find a time that you all can meet regularly or an event that you do regularly as you are forming your group. Even start with one person and add women to the group as you go. Weekly coffee, walks, wine, dinner, or whatever common thread you might have will work—but regular meet ups are key here.

- Consider naming your tribe. A longtime friend of mine named her tribe The Cats. They are hilarious lifelong friends and soul mates, and it makes me smile to see them together. This is key. Naming your tribe can make the group special—we like to belong to something that is special, and this is a way to make that happen.

- Ask for support from your spouse or family to allow you to put time and energy into the process of forming this group. Even though you are undoubtedly stretched to the max, this process and group will give you more openness in your life and broaden your success in so many areas. It's worth asking for help creating your tribe.

Keep in mind that your tribe will have a huge influence on every aspect of your life, from your level of happiness to your personal growth and even your level of income. So, choose wisely. The members of your tribe are your allies on your life's journey. When you create and expand your tribe, look for those who will lift you up, help you grow, recharge your batteries, inspire you, celebrate with you, and kick you in the butt when you need it most. The important thing to remember is that this needs to be reciprocal for it to grow into a beautiful circle of support. All members have responsibilities when it comes to the tribe, including you. So, give back to your tribe, and encourage others to do the same.

Now that you have all the tips and tools you need at your disposal, go out and make your tribe, or if you have a tribe now, be more deliberate about fine-tuning it. Add others who will make it better, or gently remove those who are not supporting the tribal goals. Your mind, work, and mission in life will thank you. I can promise you that.

Brilliant Tribe Success Story

Paula was a beautiful powerhouse of a woman working from home as a human resource consultant and was as involved as anyone could be with her kids' activities, the local school board, and all the other responsibilities around her home. Paula was one of the most "can-do" women I have ever met. She can fix a leaking toilet, build a greenhouse, tend to her children's needs, chaperone field trips, and keep up with the laundry.

She was fortunate to have a stable job that allowed her to work from home, but a problem had arisen in her life, and she was feeling extremely isolated and depressed when she came to see me. We went to work on correcting the myriad of perimenopausal deficiencies that were present, including a raging estrogen level, rock-bottom testosterone level, little to no morning cortisol, and low thyroid hormone. We helped clean up her diet, and she started daily cardio, which helped her drop 15 pounds of body fat and improve her mood and overall well-being. But she was still feeling isolated, lonely, and depressed.

We talked at length about what could be causing her to feel "unfulfilled." She admitted that she missed the days when she could meet up with friends, take a spontaneous day trip to the beach with a girlfriend, or just go have pizza and a beer with a group of people she enjoyed being around. She admitted she had not had this in her life since her college days.

HER GAME PLAN INCLUDED THE FOLLOWING:

Spending 90 days searching for at least two women she could count on for regular meeting times to have lunch, coffee, or drinks. These needed to be women she felt would: make her laugh, talk honestly with her, understand her need to work and raise a family, be fun and available, support her when she needed it, and be there for her to lighten the load.

We agreed she would notify me of who she found at the end of the 90 days to keep her accountable, but it turns out she didn't need that long. Only 30 days later, Paula called me and told me she had found three new friends that fit all of these criteria and that two of them had been there all along—she just had not put any effort into meeting with them. She asked for them to meet her at least twice a month for dinner and to support each other and that they had already met once. She said finding these women and texting, emailing, and meeting that one time had already helped her feel better; it was truly the missing piece in her life that she so desperately needed. She was eager to go on creating a full tribe and could now see why strong women need other strong women surrounding them.

She has now gone on to incorporate more members into her tribe, and nearly every woman in the group has equally benefitted from Paula's efforts. She said to me recently, "Nisha, you know, the interesting thing is that we spend so much time making everything and everyone around us better, healthier, and happier, and yet we crazy busy women often do nothing to maintain our internal need for companionship, connection, and support when that is really what helps us stay strong."

The *New* Brilliant You . . . Built to Last: How to Use Your Mind-set, Intentions, Positivity, and Awareness to Sustain a Better You

"Be thankful for what you have, and you'll end up having more. If you concentrate on what you don't have, you will never have enough."

—OPRAH WINFREY

How can you be sure you're not unconsciously perpetuating negativity in your life? Use the following quiz to gauge your personal level of negative energy.

QUIZ: ARE YOU KNEE-DEEP IN NEGATIVITY?

1. Do you complain? All the time or even just sometimes? Y/N

2. Do you often discuss what's wrong in the world more than what's right? This includes the terrible weather, horrible traffic, idiotic government, lousy economy, and stupid in-laws. Y/N

3. Do you criticize too much? Finding faults in every little thing or even just certain people? Y/N

4. Are you attracted to drama and disaster (for example, answer no if you can unglue yourself from the TV when there's a news story of a disaster and can avoid getting involved in the lives of dysfunctional celebrities)? Y/N

5. Do you blame others or yourself—either all of the time or in certain situations? Y/N

6. Do you believe you have no control over the things that happen in your life? Y/N

7. Do you often feel like a victim? Y/N

8. Are you only grateful when things finally start going right for you instead of being grateful for what is? Y/N

9. Do you feel as though things are happening to you, as opposed to happening through you? Y/N

If you said yes to four or more of the above, you are heading down the wrong path.

If you said yes to more than six of the above, you are probably a bit of a negative Nelly whose mind has been trapped in a long-term funk. It is time to reset your thoughts, words, and mind-set, because frankly it's impossible to be the most brilliant version of yourself when you are negative all the time.

THE BACKGROUND OF BLAMING

These days, brilliant, busy women find themselves caught up in negativity, worry, constant complaining, and blaming. They see these bad habits as ways of gaining some sort of control over stressful situations. The negativity and worry within us eventually attract relationships, experiences, and health issues that are riddled with even more negativity. And every negative experience gets in the way of our healthy, loving, abundant life.

Negative emotions stop us from creating the life we want. The negativity of anger, resentment, hurt, judgment, disappointment, self-doubt, and guilt stop the flow of positive living dead in its tracks. I get it. We all have bad days. They are inevitable. And the more successful you are, the more that can go wrong. The reality is that you have a choice to make—each minute of each day—as to how you react to any given situation, no matter how significant or insignificant it is. Taking responsibility for your own negativity can be the first step to becoming the brilliant you.

To do this, you must become aware of these negative reactions. Fear resides underneath this negativity—fear of rejection, fear of being loved, fear of being alone, fear of not being good enough, fear of not being approved, fear of failure, fear of death, and so on. Someone's actions or words can take us to a place of fear, and the hurt we experience distracts us and we are unable to face the fear head-on. If we blame the other person or situation instead of seeing the truth, we will continue to bring this fear into our lives.

The negativity, disrespect, and judgment in our relationships can be quite revealing about how we feel about ourselves. The struggles in our relationships with others show us that we don't fully accept, respect, appreciate, or realize that we are good enough, smart enough, or worthy of everything we want. We don't have to have a relationship with critical and judgmental people, but they may be in our life because we are critical and judgmental.

Blaming others and seeing them as wrong, unworthy, unintelligent, or unlovable stops us from facing the certain aspects in ourselves that we may need to work on. Blaming, judgment, projecting, withdrawing, tip-toeing around situations, or sweeping things under the rug are all tools we use to distract ourselves from fear. Our negative thoughts continue to cover it up. These fears then lay dormant in our memory cells, like a low-lying infection, eventually becoming a disease in our physical body, waiting for something to happen to bring them back up and make us sick.

STAY POSITIVE

Positive thinking is a good thing, but it is also considered a soft and fluffy term and is easy to dismiss. In the real world, it rarely carries the same weight as words like *work ethic* or *persistence*. But that may be changing.

Research is beginning to reveal that positive thinking is about much more than simply being happy or displaying an upbeat attitude.[41] Positive thoughts can create real value in your life and help you build skills that last much longer than a smile. The impact of positive thinking on your work, your health, and your life is being studied by people like Barbara Fredrickson.

Fredrickson is a positive psychology researcher at the University of North Carolina, and she published a landmark paper that provides surprising insights about positive thinking and its impact on your skills.[42] Her work is among the most referenced and cited in her field, and it is surprisingly useful in everyday life. So let's talk about Fredrickson's discovery and what it means for you.

---

41 Barbara L. Fredrickson, "Updated Thinking on Positivity Ratios," *American Psychologist* 68 no.9 (2013): 814–822, doi: 10.1037/a0033584.

42 Barbara L. Fredrickson, "Positive Emotions Broaden and Build," in E. Ashby Plant and P. G. Devine (eds.) *Advances in Experimental Social Psychology* 47 (2013): 1–53.

What Negative Thoughts Do to Your Brain

Play along with me for a moment. Let's say that you're walking to your car late at night, and all of the sudden you realize someone just stepped out of a dark alley and is right behind you. When something like this happens, your brain registers a negative emotion—in this case, it's fear.

Researchers have long known that negative emotions cause you to take specific actions.[43] When that intruder steps into your path, for example, you run. The rest of the world doesn't matter. You are focused entirely on the possible problem behind you, the fear it creates, and how you can get away from it as quickly as possible.

In other words, negative emotions narrow your mind and focus your thoughts. At that same moment, you might have the option to scream, jump into someone else's car, turn around and punch them in the face, or try to call for emergency help, but your brain often ignores all of those options, because they seem irrelevant when an intruder is right behind you.

This is a useful instinct if you're trying to save your life, but in ordinary, everyday situations, that narrow focus can be a huge hindrance. The problem is that your brain is still programmed to respond to any negative emotions in the same way—by shutting off the outside world and limiting your options.

For example, when you're in a fight with someone, your anger and emotion might consume you to the point where you can't think about anything else. Or when you are stressed out about everything you have to get done, you may find it hard to start because you're paralyzed by how long your to-do list has become. Similarly, if you feel bad about not exercising or eating healthy, often all you can think about is how little willpower you have, how lazy you are, and how you don't have any motivation.

In each case, your brain closes off from the outside world and focuses

43 Barbara L. Fredrickson, Michael A. Cohn, Kimberly A. Coffey, Jolynn Pek, and Sandra M. Finkel, "Open Hearts Build Lives: Positive Emotions, Induced Through Loving-Kindness Meditation, Build Consequential Personal Resources," *Journal of Personality and Social Psychology* 95, no. 5(2008), doi: 10.1037/a0013262.

on the negative emotions of fear, anger, and stress—as it did with the stranger in the alley. Negative emotions prevent your brain from seeing the other options and choices that are available to you. It's your survival instinct. Now, let's compare this to what positive emotions do to your brain.

The Effects of Positive Thinking on the Brain

Positive emotions have tremendous, long-lasting effects on the brain. According to research, people who focus on positive events throughout the day naturally identify far more solutions to problems than those who are negative.[44] In other words, those who experience emotions like joy, contentment, and love will see more opportunities in their lives. Positive emotions broaden your sense of possibility and open your mind to more options.

In addition, a positive mind-set is not only good for you in the moment; it also has a lasting effect. Being positive allows you to build skills that will continue to help you throughout your life. It creates more possibilities for you down the road, and a positive mind-set allows you to fully appreciate the big picture and be the most brilliant version of yourself.

Negative and Positive Energy

Positive energy has a variety of meanings, depending on who you ask, but it is not well defined in modern psychology. In its simplest usage, positive energy is thought of as a bundle of desirable attributes. As such, a person with positive energy is one who is enthusiastic, empathic, cheerful, optimistic, courteous, generous, kind, and open to new experiences—a

---

44 Ibid.

great person. While it would be great if there were some magic recipe for positive energy (besides being a perfect person), we need to be realistic and discuss how we can make this a reality.

We tend to perceive negative energy as something other people have. But did you know that negativity can be so ingrained that it goes unnoticed? Think about it. Have you ever been around someone who does nothing but spew negativity, complaints, and injustices, barfing out one worry statement after the next to the point where you feel as if you have been slimed with all of their bad stuff? You probably left that interaction never wanting to talk to them again.

Well, here's the bad news. You know that like attracts like, right? Positive people are drawn to positive energy; negative people are drawn to negative energy. And studies show that being negative requires *more* energy than being positive.[45] Why in the world would we ever choose to have low energy and put forth more effort by being negative? It's so much easier to be positive. It seems silly if you ask me. Instead, focus on the positive so you can create more good things in your life and save your energy for cultivating experiences that you truly want to.

The Power of Self-Talk

In case you are starting to think that you might be more negative than you realized, I want to shed some light on the impact self-talk has on your life. Studies reveal that 80 percent of self-talk is negative.[46] That's a pretty high number, but it doesn't have to be. Everything you do is positively or negatively affected by self-talk and your inner thoughts. That's why getting rid of negative self-talk is one of the most basic actions we must do to remain successful and happy.

---

45 Barbara Fredrickson and Marcial Losada, "Positive Affect and the Complex Dynamics of Human Flourishing," *American Psychologist* 60, no. 7 (2005): 678–686, doi: 10.1037/0003-066x.60.7.678.

46 Ben Martin, "Challenging Negative Self-Talk," Psych Central, https://psychcentral.com/lib/challenging-negative-self-talk/.

I remember when I first started working with women in the gynecology office and quickly noticed that so many of my most favorite patients were those who exuded positivity. I wanted to talk to them, be with them, and help them. At the same time, I noticed that my chronically negative patients seemed to develop more and more ailments, almost like strange gynecological issues that didn't make sense, and their hormones were often off balance even with treatment.

Early on, I started asking some of my patients to write down every thought that came into their brain for two to three consecutive days. Several of my patients followed through with this and brought the list in for me to see. It was awful. I'd never seen such intense negativity. This was a huge wake-up call for me personally and professionally. Nearly every statement and thought, verbal or nonverbal, was negative. From the minute they got out of bed, they were saying things like "I am so fat," "I am late again," "I have no time to exercise," "I slept terrible last night," "I am so tired, so sick, so stressed, so exhausted, so brain-dead," "I am sick of this house being a mess; why doesn't anyone do anything around here," "why am I the only one doing anything," and on and on.

But the really interesting thing about these lists is that out of the hundred or so thoughts they wrote down, fewer than 5 in a 24-hour period of time were positive. So in the group that I asked to do this, nearly 95 percent of the thoughts they had were negative and in fact pretty damaging. But imagine what we could do if we said as many positive things to ourselves throughout the day.

The Health Consequences of Negativity

Negativity plays a key role in burnout. The thing to remember here is that negative emotions are bad for your health, especially if you allow them to multiply and consume your every waking moment. Left untreated, negativity can lead to depression, ruined relationships, alcohol and substance abuse, financial problems, health problems, body pain, anxiety, bad decision making, and accelerated aging. Ultimately, negativity breeds even more negativity in your life. The idea that your emotions impact your health and the development of disease is not new. Even the conservative Centers for Disease Control and Prevention (CDC) has stated that 85 percent of all diseases appear to have an emotional element (though the actual percentage is likely to be even higher).

And once you get into a pattern of negative thinking, it can be difficult to break. These unpleasant feelings end up becoming routine. Your attitude, whether positive or negative, has a dramatic effect in every area of your life. Everyone gets angry, but having chronic feelings of depression, anger, guilt, condemnation, and low self-esteem are all lethal toxins that ultimately damage our health. Unfortunately, the issue is that anger triggers the fight-or-flight stress response, pumping our brilliant minds with chemicals needed to fuel this intense emotion and bleeding us dry of the very energy and stamina we need to manage our busy lives.

The real truth is that nearly every time we burst out in anger, it is completely unnecessary. We can't afford this negative thought process if we are ultimately going to be successful and live longer. This is why it is not only necessary that we manage our diet, sleep, hormones, and supplements, but we must also tend to our thoughts and emotions so we have more stamina and can stay in the game.

The long-term consequences of emotional upset and chronic negativity most often include the following:

- Anxiety

- Depression

- High blood pressure

- Skin problems

- Accelerated aging

- Headaches

- Digestive imbalances

- Heart attack

- Stroke

- Cancer

- Suppressed immune system

- Weight gain or low metabolism

It turns out that the majority of the physical symptoms negativity produces can be blamed on the weakening of your veins and arteries. Lashing out or internalizing anger via unprocessed regret, negativity, bitterness, or fear are all emotions that fuel stress hormones that surge through your body and injure blood vessel linings. Bruce Wright, MD, says lashing out in anger can make stress hormones surge and injure blood vessel linings, tripling your risk of a heart attack.[47]

These feelings affect the body as well. Research points to the fact that being chronically angry, negative, or fearful can move you closer to what you are afraid of or angry about[48]—not exactly what you want to be doing in your successful, brilliant life. We want more: more brilliance, success, happiness, positivity, and lightness. To accomplish this, we need to move away from the things that are preventing us from being well, aging better, and ultimately being so much happier.

This is difficult for brilliant women to do because we are busy, driven,

47 Don Colbert, *Deadly Emotions: Understand the Mind-Body-Spirit Connection That Can Heal or Destroy You* (Nashville, TN: Thomas Nelson, 2006).

48 Ibid.

and focused, with an over-the-top work ethic that sees us run right over the tops of others, often expecting them to keep up and perform like us. This is only one of the situations in which brilliant women can fester anger, frustration, resentment, and further emotional distress. This is why I suggest you work on overcoming your emotional barriers first in your quest to combat burnout. Whether they're current issues or past issues, they must be dealt with to live your best, fullest life. Trust me, I get that this is hard. I still have and continue to work on my own emotional demons. Everyone has them. But I also can attest to how vital it is that you confront them. Today.

Here's a tip I'm going to give you for this (and frankly, this is probably the most important point of this chapter). Every three months, stop and ask yourself, "Am I better now than I was?" It is critical that you answer yes to this every time. If you are not getting better, then by definition you are getting worse, since nothing stays the same. There are a host of techniques that can be used to calm yourself, regroup, reframe, move out destructive negative thought patterns, and lighten your emotional load to ultimately create a sense of inner peace. The best rule is to find one that works for you. Whether it's conventional or alternative doesn't matter. As long as it's making you better, do it and keep using it to stop and reroute your negative state.

ACHIEVING ULTIMATE HAPPINESS

To be successful, one of the first things we must learn to do is control our minds. Our mind is the central place from which we plan and execute all the necessary actions for success. This means you should be paying attention to the thoughts that occupy your mind at all times, or as much as you can. Doing so will allow you to realize what is happening in your head as well as what triggers your negativity.

For sure, success leads to happiness. Winning a tennis match does it for me. Other common examples might be landing a better job, finding someone you love, or feeling the pride of putting together a leadership team or business model that is wildly successful. All of these things bring joy, contentment, and a sense of accomplishment. But it's rarely that simple. We often assume that happiness will follow success. But that ends up always being the next success, so it becomes unattainable.

I will be the first to admit that I am pathologically driven to reach beyond what is remotely normal. I have been guilty of putting off happiness until I achieve the next greatest thing. But happiness *now* is essential to success. Happiness is a precursor to success as well as a result of it. This is what researchers define as an "upward spiral" that occurs with positive, happy, content people. They look at things differently, and they seek out new skills to help them stay mentally and emotionally centered. And happiness is the result, which nearly always leads to more success. It is a like a chain reaction. So let's talk about how we can get this chain reaction started.

Positivity

Positive thinking and a positive mind-set are goals you must commit yourself to. If you're reading this, you most likely need to work on this. It's essential to your longevity. Being positive takes a hell of a lot of work and, for most of us, does not come naturally, especially when we are living in a world that is negative and full of complications and roadblocks. I'll be honest: Sometimes I just want to hide in a cave and never come out because everything feels as if it is falling apart. These times require us to immediately pull out our internal tools for dealing with this.

The following quick-fix regrouping tools can be absolutely invaluable when you are going through especially trying times:

- The three-minute rule: When someone says something that makes you want to rip their head off, wait three minutes (or for God's sake 30 seconds if you can't do any more) and then answer. This could require leaving the room, changing the subject, or asking for some time to come up with a solution.

- Daily meditation once or twice per day with or without prayer

- Deep breathing

- In the moments of total breakdown, find three things that you are thankful for, no matter what.

- In moments of anger directed at a person, say, "I love you. I forgive you. I am thankful for you" (even if you are not). And then come up with two to three things that are positive about this person or situation. (This is a virtual marriage saver!)

- In the moments of extreme frustration, take yourself to a place much worse and then thank the angels above that you are not there.

- Journal daily about things you are thankful for: This is one of the greatest and easiest ways to refocus and get yourself out of a negative mind-set.

- Go out for a walk. This is one of my personal favorites. I do this often at the office. When I feel like my head is going to blow right off my shoulders, I take a minute and leave, walk up the sidewalk, breathe, look at the beautiful trees (Oregon is so wonderful in that way), and say:

  - "Do not be afraid."

  - "Let this go."

- "Do not attach yourself to this anger."

- "What can I see in this situation that is good?"

- "Is this really happening or have I created this in my mind?"

- "What can I do right now to move in a different direction?"

- "How can I best be a leader to those who admire me right now?"

- "How do I know this is true?"

- "Is this situation worth my current reaction to it?"

- If you are outside regrouping, look at a tree or bench or something else stationary, and mentally leave your anger there. It sounds weird, but try it. Drop it on the bench or tree. Dispose of it. See it leaving your body. It works.

- If you can't leave a situation that is escalating, then:

  - Start breathing deep from your belly.

  - Force yourself to smile.

  - Look at the person or group or situation and imagine a huge, golden sunshine like rays pouring down from above right into the group or situation. Keep focusing on this ray of light, and while you are listening, focus on the positive, beautiful energy flowing into the situation.

  - Take your hand and run it down the front of your body, as if you were cutting the cord between you and the situation or the person. This will help you mentally disconnect from the situation. The alternative is mentally replaying it over and over again in your mind for hours. Instead, cut the cord and be done with it.

People do stupid things, don't pay attention, are disrespectful, often don't care, and are caught up in their own suffering—so cut it all a bit of a break and move lightly through this world, getting the best of things and leaving the worst for someone else to attach to. It's not for you, brilliant babe!

IT'S ALL ABOUT BALANCE

Even I forget the importance of balance at times. Life is crazy, and some days you have to focus on getting the important things done, whether you're dealing with kids, your partner, or your job. The important thing is that you come back to a place of balance and make sure that your life is not *all* work. You must be sure that you make time for yourself. Turn off your computer, be creative, play, watch a mindless TV show, hike, get outside, and travel. Making time for these things is incredibly important. It is about taking care of all parts of *you*! Remember, though, balance is an ongoing process. Balance is not about being calm all the time, but rather practicing daily principles of balance so you are constantly aware of where you are in each moment and how you feel about what is happening on any given day or week, allowing you to adjust as needed.

These days, we all seem to be "on call" when we are not physically at work. This means we are "on" during most of our waking hours and trying to take care of things. With phones, computers, texting, and the like, we often never turn off. This is a model that women (especially us brilliant women) cannot sustain. Even if you are not displaying any obvious side effects from this now, trust me, you will eventually.

You may feel as if you don't have much control over being "on" all the time. In that case, it is important to regularly ask yourself, "In what ways am I bringing enjoyment or joy into my life?" This particular question cannot be answered by saying, "I work." We have to use both sides of our brain to fulfill all aspects of what we need in our lives to be complete brilliant women. Too much work will destroy your sense of balance and lead you to negativity and resentment. Some suggestions on how to avoid blazing the trail to burnout and how you can bring balance back into your life are listed below:

- **Build some "no fly time" into each day.** Is there a possibility that from 5:00 to 7:00 a.m. you could only either work out, meditate, or get outside? This means no emails, phone calls, or text messages during this time. Is it possible that at 6:00 p.m. you turn it all off? Can you talk to your employees, coworkers, or boss and tell them you need to shut down at a certain time and to only reach out if there's an emergency? Building downtime into your schedule will save your brain and your nervous system from a lot of long-term damage.

- **Get rid of any unnecessary activities you are doing that zap your energy.** So many women waste time on activities, functions, meetings, and volunteering that make no difference in their life and add absolutely no value. We also have a tendency to rant about situations that will never change. This is something you have to stop doing, because it is precious time you are wasting that could be spent with things you love to do or should be doing that *do* add value to your life. Consider spending less time on what adds no value (social media or browsing the internet or volunteer work that you do *not* need to be doing or are not passionate about). Instead, add in some things that add value to your life and your career.

- **Find one thing every year that you want to master, and start planning time to do it each week.** Some examples of this include horseback riding (my personal favorite), learning a new language (painful but useful), going to a fitness group, taking up a craft that you have always wanted to learn, or becoming an expert in wine, cooking, or something creative that allows you to expand what you are interested in. If you have no interests besides work, kids, and home, pick the thing that might be something you like (but keep it simple), and then do it weekly for at least an hour. If you are a stay-at-home mom, find ways to do some things on your own time that do not include the kids. This is vital for women who feel stuck and dissatisfied with what they are doing the majority of the week.

- **Incorporate daily movement.** We have spent enough time over the course of this book on the benefits of getting your body moving. Just do it—your entire being will thank you for it (and so will your kids and partner).

- **Set priorities, and write them down.** I personally love Peter Drucker's leadership for business books. He talks a lot about setting goals and doing the most important ones first. Too often, we do the easy stuff first, and then our entire day is wasted, and the most important projects are left for later. Attack these projects first thing in the morning every day, when you are sharp and clear. The most difficult part is figuring out what is the most important thing for you to focus on at any given moment. Always ask yourself what your priority is for any given day. Is checking your email or Facebook more important than calling your mother? Is getting your shoes on and heading outside more important than sleeping in another hour? Is talking to your best friend or texting for three hours per day more important than hammering out that work project in silence for three hours? Your number-one priority is a moving target, and you need to be on task. If you get off-track, regroup and tackle one thing that day instead of 50. You must focus and get the top priorities taken care of so you can then move on to things later in the day or night that nourish your soul.

- **Set short- and long-term goals.** Set goals in every aspect of your life: personally, professionally, emotionally, and spiritually. You should have daily goals, weekly goals, and longer-term goals and aspirations. Who do you want to be? What are you striving for? What and how can you best use your gifts on this earth? What legacy do you ultimately want to leave behind? Make goals for your role as a mother, wife, and friend and write them down. Make sure they are specific, and write them down in a book that you keep with you. There are many apps and books on how to write effective goals, but the important thing is that you start doing it. This is so vital for balance and for your soul.

- **Understand that accomplishments and failures are part of balance.** Remember to look honestly at your setbacks and failures as well as your successes. Most of us have daily doses of both, but we may not have time to pay attention and learn from them. If, however, you are overfocusing on failures or setbacks, then begin the process by considering your successes (even if they are little) that you have. Keep adjusting as necessary. If you are overfocusing on the negative, ask yourself why. Are you afraid of success, do you think you don't deserve it, or are you beating yourself up because you are tired and need to be rejuvenated with the things in your life you love doing? It is important to ask yourself these questions. Look at your failures and learn from them, learn about how to avoid them, how this avoidance is protecting you, and how you can avoid them next time. Look at your successes and ask yourself, "How did that happen?" "How can I bring more of this into my life?" Remember, you are always in transition. Our busy lives are not static, and you need to learn to float through life without getting stuck. Being in balance is a process, and as Mindy Bacharach said, "Balance is the process of holding something(s) steady during change."[49]

---

49 https://www.mindybacharach.com/blog/.

So now we are at the end of our time together. I can't tell you how happy I am that you stuck with me and got this far. This has been a fun journey for me, and I truly hope that it has been for you, too. I am going to leave you with a fast-track plan for further positivity development and want you to always remember that whatever happens in the mind will be reflected in your body, so keep it positive. We have more power within us than we can imagine, and most of us never tap into it.

It's time to take your brilliance to another level. If you get stuck along the way, consider talking to me directly. It is my job after all, and together we can get you into the best place ever! Your brilliant life is my mission, and I want this world to be filled with healthy, powerful, happy women who make it a better place to be.

FAST-TRACK PLAN FOR ULTIMATE SUCCESS AND HAPPINESS

Now that you have come this far with your newfound enlightenment on moving forward with more consistent positive thoughts, pushing away the negativity and leaning in, creating "down-time" for your mind and soul, let me spoon-feed you with a few more tips on reaching a new brilliant YOU height that will for sure prove to open you up and be fun in the process!

- **Meditate regularly.** Research shows that those who meditate daily for even ten minutes (mindless sitting or any other form of mental relaxation) immediately discover increased mindfulness, a sense of purpose, more social support, and even decreased illness. Meditation also increases productivity and decreases stress. It improves health, relationships, and helps people find a connection to nature and the universe. Practice the same meditation every day for a month to receive the maximum benefit and to effectively change the thought pathways in your brain.

- **Start playing more.** Schedule time to play. We schedule meetings, conference calls, weekly events, and other responsibilities into our daily calendars, so why not schedule time to play? When was the last time you carved out time for nothing more than a fun activity? You can't tell me being happy and playful is less important than your weekly meetings. Put it on the calendar.

- **Understand that to be successful you have to work your butt off.** Every single person who is highly successful will tell you how much work it is. Give yourself permission to smile at this fact and know it is part of the process. It's okay to work hard. However, it's not okay to complain about it and set yourself in a downward spiral of negativity. This path is part of what you have chosen to be good at, so don't be bitter.

- **Be your own inner coach.** To be successful, choose your thoughts wisely and deliberately. When you find yourself in the midst of fear, anger, resentment, or defeatist thinking, it's time to regroup and realize that you are on the wrong path. Develop a way to recognize when what you are saying is negative, and immediately turn it off. When challenges surface in business, you might experience a loss of control over emotions and thoughts. To remain optimistic, discipline your mind to stay clear of catastrophic thoughts and the slippery slope of anxiety. Those of you who have operated in the negative for years will likely at first not recognize when this negativity sets in, or you will try to rationalize it by saying you are just talking to a friend or venting some frustrations. But that's not really the case. Get rid of the negative. It's infectious and not healthy, and without attending to it you will only bring more negativity into your life. This is not good for women who need to make a difference in this world. Instead, focus on solutions.

- **Don't jump to conclusions.** In this pattern of negative thinking, you assume that you know what everyone is thinking, and it's normally negative in regard to yourself. This may involve concluding that another person is reacting negatively to you without concrete evidence or even validating this with them. Often what we think is happening is only a slice of it, but because we have blown it up to be such a monolithic, negative drama in our brains, we see that tiny slice as way more than it actually is. Keep in mind this thought principle of Hanlon's razor: "Never attribute to malice that which can be adequately explained by stupidity. Never make assumptions. Always check out your perceptions first before jumping to conclusions."

- **Create a positive impression on those around you every day.** To reach your peak potential on the climb to success, be driven, goal oriented, honest, and bold, but more importantly be happy and enjoyable to work for and with. Your personal vibe can either repel people or draw them in. When you carry an attitude of excitement and vigor, this transfers to those around you and increases business morale. If your attitude is gregarious, infectious, and all about living life to its fullest, then you will seem to have unlimited potential. People love this and are naturally attracted to winners. So *be* a winner and a leader that other women and men admire.

- **Find something that feeds your soul.** Connecting with your spiritual self will nurture your soul—and, by proxy, your business. The deeper the connection you feel to the purpose of your business and life, the more you will experience it. Finding purpose in what you do and knowing you are using the gifts you were given will pay you back beyond belief. Practice nourishing your soul daily in any way that is right for you, and above all make sure to know your purpose on this earth.

- **Keep it light.** Find the humor in life as you continue being the brilliant woman you are. This will not only lower your stress, but it will also create energy around you that others want a piece of, including business associates, family, and friends. Find a way to laugh every day, as many times a day as you can.

- **Believe you will succeed.** To be successful, you must understand that there are only two things you truly have control over: your thoughts and your feelings. That's pretty much it. Exude positivity in your work ethic and in your interactions with others. A brilliant woman must have determination, resilience, and a great attitude. You will kill it if you understand this, and you will be happier for it. Dominate your world by harnessing the power of your positive inner self. This practice is the basis for nearly every successful person to date. Choose to attract what you want by harnessing your attitude about success; you will find that success more attainable.

- **Live every day with purpose.** Every day is a new opportunity. Live every day with intention and don't let life just happen. Instead, live your life on purpose and with true meaning so happiness can naturally flow in and out of you. Tell yourself you love your life, you love your job, you love your family, and so on, and then remind yourself why you do. Tell yourself that you are here to make a difference in as many people's lives as possible. You are here to use your brilliance to make the world better. Choose the roads you want to travel, and say no to the ones that cause you anxiety. You don't need that in your life. And don't be a passenger. Get in the driver's seat, and make your life have as much meaning and joy as humanly possible. It's worth the ride.

- **Begin the mantras for success.** No matter how successful you are (or hopefully will be one day), you will need to choose your daily mantras and then dedicate yourself to them. The interesting thing about brilliant women is that everyone around them knows they are strong, courageous, energetic, and powerful, but the reality is that we are still human and need to be supported, loved, and surrounded by those who will help us. Thus, in the process of finding happiness, we must not only ask for help, but we must also practice our mantras of who we want to be and the positivity we want to exude. This is a powerful practice that has tremendous results. If you are not mantra-ing, you are forfeiting huge benefits. So, get your cards out, write your mantras on them, place them everywhere, and say your powerful words every day. If you need some examples to get you started, here are the ones I use:

  - I am worth it.

  - I am smart.

  - I am lovable.

  - I am unique.

  - I am happy.

  - I attract healthy relationships.

  - I enjoy health in my life, mind, body, and spirit.

  - I attract abundance and prosperity.

  - I love my life.

  - I am connected to my life's purpose.

- **Be grateful.** It's easy to become consumed with all the things that are going wrong in your life or all the losses you've suffered. But this only serves to depress your mood and keep you stuck. Instead, look at how far you've come and at what *is* working well in your life. It may be as simple as having food in your belly and a roof over your head. Being grateful for what you have in the here and now helps give you a healthier perspective and opens the doors for receiving even more good in your life. It also relieves stress, reduces depression, reframes your thinking, and opens up a whole world of possibilities. So hop on the gratitude train. You'll be glad you did.

- **Pay it forward.** This may be the most important thing I can teach you. Once your life starts to turn around, it will gather momentum in a big way. It may take time, but if you follow the right steps, things will improve. And when they do, you may want to think about paying it forward. Giving back in a spirit of gratefulness is incredibly fulfilling. You may want to donate money to a worthy cause or give your time, energy, or talent to others who are just starting out or need your assistance. It doesn't matter what you do. Paying it forward helps cultivate a sense of gratefulness and comes with its own higher rewards. You can turn your life around and, in doing so, inspire countless others to do the same. If that's not brilliant, then I don't know what is.

APPENDIX A

Supplements for Stress and Adrenal Function

- **A.M. and P.M. STRESS Supplements.** Both of these supplements are used to re-create an optimal cortisol pattern. The a.m. stress supplement contains L-tyrosine, ashwagandha, Korean ginseng, and other botanicals to help optimize the cortisol during the day for energy, focus, stamina, and assistance managing daytime stressors. The p.m. stress supplements contain phosphorylated serine that suppresses cortisol at night to help you shut down your busy brain and sleep deeply.

- **Adrenal Cortex Extracts.** Utilizing adrenal cortex glandular extracts help regulate daytime cortisol when levels are very low, thus negatively affecting your ability to get out of bed and function at an optimal level.

- **Vitamin C Concentrated Powder.** Using high-dose ascorbic acid (vitamin C) will help promote the needed adrenal support to manufacture cortisol. One half to one teaspoon of vitamin C powder (2,000-4,000 mg) with food in your morning water bottle and again in the afternoon can be instrumental in getting the necessary energy-boosting daytime cortisol.

- **B Complex Sublingual Drops.** All B vitamins (better in combination rather than alone) support the entire adrenal system. This particular high-powered sublingual B complex is used under the tongue daily after breakfast or lunch.

- **Clary Sage.** Aromatherapy uses the power of scent to calm the mind and reduce anxiety. Your olfactory system affects the part of your brain that regulates emotion. When used as an aromatherapy protocol, clary sage can help alleviate stress by inducing a sense of well-being. This essential oil can be used at night or during the day as a scent you can smell throughout the day. You can also use it in a carrier oil by rubbing it into your wrists or temples.

*All supplements are available at BalanceDocs.com or at your favorite reputable health food store.

Supplements to Regulate Estrogen Metabolism

- **DIM.** This supplement improves estrogen metabolism and helps to prevent estrogen dominance in men and women.

- **Zinc.** This supplement improves the hormone pathways for men and women while keeping estrogen in a nondominant state in the body.

- **Progesterone Topical Cream.** This unique and powerful plant-based cream is a slam dunk for estrogen dominance and the side effects of it. Use this topically at bedtime for younger or older women to reduce breast tenderness, ovarian cysts, PMS, depression, and anxiety issues.

*All supplements listed above are available at BalanceDocs.com or at your favorite reputable health food store.

APPENDIX C

Supplements for Mood Support

- **MOOD Rebalance.** This supplement has a combination of amino acids and botanicals formulated to boost the brain chemicals serotonin and GABA. This supplement works the first time it is taken. Additionally, this supplement improves sleep, while reducing anxiety and cravings.

- **Progesterone Topical Cream.** This can be used nightly or during PMS.

- **B Complex Drops or Capsules.** To be taken sublingually once or twice daily.

*All supplements listed above are available at BalanceDocs.com or at your favorite reputable health food store.

APPENDIX D

Supplements for Optimal Sleep

- **SLEEP Rebalance.** This high-potency supplement is formulated to support all sleep brain chemicals and to help induce deep sleep while helping to calm your nervous system. It is powerful and can be helpful while weaning off prescription sleep aids.

- **Melatonin.** Using higher dosages of melatonin when needed can be necessary to break the neurological patterns that develop over time. This can be used with the above sleep supplement from BalanceDocs.com.

- **Pregnenolone.** This supplement supports most of the hormones and stress system downstream. It can be very helpful to break a long-standing insomnia pattern, while boosting necessary adrenal and female hormone levels naturally. This supplement is intended to be used if serum levels are deficient and for shorter periods of time.

*All supplements listed above are available at BalanceDocs.com or at your favorite reputable health food store.

APPENDIX E

Supplements to Regulate Appetite and Cravings

- **Craving.** This supplement will help boost the brain chemical norepinephrine that helps put the brakes on cravings.

- **Energy.** This supplement boosts energy (overeating happens with fatigue) while supporting the adrenal function naturally and controlling appetite.

- **Liposlim.** Stubborn-fat-be-gone! This supplement is formulated with botanicals aimed at improving fat metabolism.

- **A.M. Stress with Tyrosine.** This supplement improves focus and energy to help you stay on your new and improved eating plan without backsliding. Boosting dopamine levels with these ingredients will arrest bad habits and keep you on track with better resilience.

*All supplements listed above are available at BalanceDocs.com or at your favorite reputable health food store.

APPENDIX F

Testing Options for Female Hormones

- **Lab in a Box Serum Testing** (sent directly to your home). At Peak Medical we offer lab testing in the convenience of your own home. If you have the need for testing or are having a difficult time finding a practitioner to test and treat you, consider ordering a **Lab in a Box.** This can be taken to a local draw site and then overnighted to our lab. Once results are available, a detailed individualized plan for optimal hormone balance can be sent to you. Go to BalanceDocs. com for ordering information on Lab in a Box.

APPENDIX G

Finding a Hormone Expert

- Peak Medical Clinic and Nisha Jackson offer private hormone consultations. These can be done via phone or a private web consult utilizing lab testing and a thorough evaluation of your unique problems and concerns. These consultations can be booked online at NishaJackson.com.

- You may also find a local expert if you contact the compounding pharmacies in your area and ask for a referral to a reputable and trained hormone expert that utilizes serum testing and bioidentical hormones. Most pharmacists already know who is the best in the area.

APPENDIX H

Cleansing Jump-start Diet for Fat Loss and Adrenal Reset

The following is a great diet to jump-start your weight loss and reset your adrenals.

BREAKFAST

Lean protein: Eat 14–21 grams of lean protein (2–3 egg whites, for example, is great). Rotate proteins daily or consider a protein shake with 21 grams of protein, unsweetened coconut water, and ¼ cup raspberries or a super-green shake with protein.

Green veggies: A handful of spinach or broccoli in the omelet works great (or choose any green veggie to eat in the a.m.).

Good fats: Avocado (1/2) or 5–7 nuts or 2 teaspoons of chia seeds, and 1 tablespoon of coconut oil with the egg-omelet

Low-sugar fruit: Sliced apple with cinnamon on it; or you can save this for a snack later

LUNCH

Lean protein: 14–21 grams (choose any lean type of protein)

Green veggies: Large green salad with chicken on top (3–4 ounces only); 1 tablespoon olive oil and apple cider vinegar dressing or Braggs amino acids drizzled on top

Good fats: Sprinkled nuts or seeds (5–7 nuts or 20–30 seeds); or consider curry chicken lettuce wraps instead of a salad

Low-sugar fruit: 1 sliced apple with cinnamon or a handful of blueberries

AFTERNOON SNACK

1 ounce of dark chocolate or another apple sliced with cinnamon

DINNER

Lean protein: 14–21 grams of lean protein; try salmon

Good veggies: Steamed veggies on the side, or make a stir-fry

Good fats: Add coconut oil to the stir-fry or sprinkle chia seeds on top of protein

Low-sugar fruit: Unsweetened applesauce heated up with cinnamon

TIPS:

• I am convinced apples are curative and help you curtail your cravings and glucose level. They are magic and might really keep the doctor away—so start eating them.

- Stop eating by 6:30 or 7:00 p.m. at the latest (only water or herbal tea after this time).

- Eat enough fat to satiate you—nuts, seeds, and good oils. Each meal should have protein, veggies, and good fats.

- Try to eat slowly, and have your foods prepared beforehand to grab and go.

- Cook chicken or proteins one to two days a week so they are ready to go.

- Set out your dinner before you leave in the morning, and consider a Crock-Pot so it is ready when you come home. Be prepared; it really helps.

- This diet is a two-week cleansing diet but can be used for months on end, as it is such a clean way of eating and supplies all the nutrients you need to stay healthy, lean, and hormonally balanced.

- After two weeks or more, you can slowly introduce high-fiber carbohydrates like small red potato, sweet potato, barley (non-flour) bread, quinoa, or brown rice. Keep portions the size of a deck of cards or less. Only have one to two servings per day. No flour or sugar, and any carbs you eat need to be high in fiber, low on the glycemic index scale, and in very small portions.

- Veggies are unlimited (especially green veggies).

- Eat four apples a day (you can substitute grapefruit, oranges, or pears for 1 of the apples per day).

- Sugar substitutes should only be stevia or xylitol.

- Read labels and keep sugars *low*.

....

Index

About the Author

NISHA JACKSON IS a hormone expert and health specialist known for providing safe and effective solutions to her patients' everyday health issues. Nisha treats stress, insomnia, depression, hormone imbalance, and other common conditions. She offers practical information to her patients in reassuring, easy-to-understand terms.

She is nationally recognized as a lecturer, motivational speaker, radio host, columnist, and author. She is also founder of many prestigious medical establishments, including Balance Docs, Inc., a national supplement corporation; Rogue Clinical Laboratories, specializing in highly sensitive hormone testing and medical training; Ventana Wellness PC, an integrative medical health clinic; and her current medical practice, Peak Medical Clinics, Inc., all dedicated to disease prevention, primary care, and hormonal health.

For Nisha, health is more about natural balance than it is pharmaceutical relief or quick-fix treatments that merely scratch the surface of wellness. In fact, her past 28 years of research and patient care have proven her right. While many physicians suggest that certain symptoms are normal, psychosomatic, or something patients must learn to live with, Nisha confidently offers patients the help and hope they want and need— but have been unable to find. Her passion for women's health began in 1990 when she realized that female patients were desperate to manage their hot flashes, PMS, low libido, menstrual irregularities, and other hormone-related symptoms. With diet, exercise, and individualized hormonal treatments, women and men who were fatigued and feeling older than their biological age started to feel their absolute best.

She has spent years formulating supplements that are the perfect balance of herbs, amino acids, vitamins, minerals, and adaptogens of the highest quality to ensure the proper control and treatment of depression, anxiety, insomnia, toxic stress, low sexual drive, and fatigue. She is a recognized bioidentical hormone trainer to physicians nationally and is the founder of The Body Analysis program, which is a medically based weight-loss program that focuses on long-term results, with an emphasis on regaining health and feeling great.

Nisha has authored two books, *The Hormone Survival Guide to Perimenopause: How to Balance Your Hormones Naturally* and *Surviving the Teenage Hormone Takeover: A Guide for Moms.*

Nisha Jackson PhD, MS, NP, HHP

NishaJackson.com
BalanceDocs.com
PeakMedicalClinic.com